Gluten
Exposed

ALSO BY PETER H. R. GREEN, M.D., AND RORY JONES, M.S.

Celiac Disease: A Hidden Epidemic

Gluten Exposed

*The Science Behind the Hype and How to
Navigate to a Healthy, Symptom-Free Life*

———

PETER H. R. GREEN, M.D.,
AND RORY JONES, M.S.

wm
WILLIAM MORROW
An Imprint of HarperCollinsPublishers

HarperCollins books may be purchased for educational, business, or sales promotional use. For information, please email the Special Markets Department at SPsales@harpercollins.com.

Chapter 7 appeared in a different form in *Celiac Disease: A Hidden Epidemic* (first ed.) by Peter H. R. Green, M.D., and Rory Jones, published by William Morrow, 2006.

FIRST EDITION

Designed by Lucy Albanese
Illustrations by Thom Graves

Names: Green, Peter H. R., author. | Jones, Rory, author.
Title: Gluten exposed : the science behind the hype and how to navigate to a healthy, symptom-free life / Peter H.R. Green, M.D. and Rory Jones, M.S.
Description: First edition. | New York, NY : William Morrow, an imprint of HarperCollinsPublishers, [2016] | Includes index.
Identifiers: LCCN 2016001185 (print) | LCCN 2016003081 (ebook) | ISBN 9780062394286 (hardback) | ISBN 9780062394293 (e-book)
Subjects: LCSH: Gluten—Health aspects—Popular works. | Gluten-free diet—Popular works. | Celiac disease—Popular works. | Self-care, Health—Popular works. | BISAC: HEALTH & FITNESS / Diets. | HEALTH & FITNESS / Nutrition. | HEALTH & FITNESS / Diseases / General.
Classification: LCC RC862.C44 G744 2016 (print) | LCC RC862.C44 (ebook) | DDC 616.3/99—dc23
LC record available at http://lccn.loc.gov/2016001185

ISBN 978-0-06-239428-6

16 17 18 19 20   RRD   10 9 8 7 6 5 4 3 2 1

Contents

A Note from the Authors

All the information in this book is based on current scientific knowledge about the effect on the body of gluten and the many foods, drugs, and supplements that we ingest. It is derived from an in-depth analysis of current medical literature, extensive clinical experience, patient and professional interviews, as well as ongoing research into the various manifestations and conditions ascribed to gluten-related disorders.

Other medical experts may have differing opinions and interpretations of the medical literature. Wherever pertinent, the authors have attempted to note conflicting points of view on key issues as well as topics that have not as yet been scientifically resolved.

Many of the peer-reviewed articles we have consulted may not be readily accessible to all readers. For this reason, we have not included footnotes for all medical facts and figures. Instead, we have listed good basic review articles and books for different subjects in the appendices.

All references to the "Center" refer to the Celiac Disease Center at Columbia University.

NOTE: This book is not a self-diagnosis manual. It is intended to generate informed patients who know what questions to ask of their physicians and how to understand the answers.

Introduction

The fewer the facts, the stronger the opinion.
—ARNOLD H. GLASOW

Simple solutions are always appealing. In the last few years, gluten has become the ultimate villain—the Wicked Witch, Darth Vader, the Joker, and Hannibal Lecter rolled into one devouring multisystem ravager. It is blamed for draining our brain, blowing up our bellies, invading our nervous system, and setting fire to our guts. A recent bestselling book claimed that: "Brain disease can be largely prevented by the choices you make in life . . ." If only it were that simple.

Almost a third of all American and UK consumers are trying to avoid gluten. By any reckoning, a significant portion of the buying public is focused on the gluten in our food supply and on their plates.

Gluten is implicated in everything from heart disease, neuralgia, sore muscles, exhaustion, "brain fog," headaches, autism, diabetes, arthritis, curious rashes, schizophrenia, dementia, weight loss, fibromyalgia, and irritable bowel syndrome to plain "it makes me feel sick-"itis. Yet most of these claims do not hold up.

In fact, it has become increasingly hard to swallow the story line written by the media as well as friends, family members, and various alternative health care professionals. The menu at this feast of confusion includes wheat and the different proteins within it, genes, germs, fungi, antibiotics, herbicides, enzymes, supplements, and anything else that travels through the intestinal tract. It is a multicourse, multisystem, increasingly nonscientific boiling pot.

Unfortunately, the food industry and general population got onto a gluten-free diet ahead of the medical community, which is now playing scientific catch-up. With the advent of the Internet, everyone has become a medical researcher. This has left room for the public to run away with ideas and point fingers at gluten as the cause for anything and everything.

Gluten has become a media-borne epidemic. **But beware: pseudoscience can be hazardous to your health.**

The Promise of Miracles

He took a grain of truth and made a loaf of baloney.
—ANONYMOUS

The majority of the information available about the effect of gluten on the body is only partly correct or almost wholly incorrect, and few people have the background or knowledge to question its accuracy. Most of the claims touted by TV hosts, books by "experts," and websites featuring the words *natural* or *doctor recommended* do not withstand scrutiny.

Which is exactly what we intend to do. Starting in the gut and working up to the brain and back, we will explore the many claims, conditions, treatments, and diets to diagnose exactly what gluten does and does not cause or cure.

In 1996, Alan Greenspan, then the Federal Reserve Board chairman, used the phrase *irrational exuberance* as a warning that the market might be overvalued. Today, this same phrase could be used to describe the emotions surrounding gluten, which is being blamed for many of the physical as well as psychological problems people suffer from. And it is becoming increasingly scientifically clear that this focus on gluten as the culprit behind "all that ails ye" is increasingly irrational.

Gluten—the "One Size Fits All" Myth

There are in fact two things, science and opinion; the
former begets knowledge, the latter ignorance.

—HIPPOCRATES

Occam's Razor is a principle utilized in medicine stating that among competing hypotheses, the hypothesis with the fewest assumptions should be selected. It seems to account for the spate of books that point to gluten as the reason behind every pain and drain in the body.

When a patient comes to the doctor—usually with a group of symptoms—the doctor needs to isolate and evaluate each issue separately, not necessarily as manifestations of the same condition. Doctors need to care for patients as a whole, and that requires a sensitive ear as well as appropriate tests and treatments. Holistic medicine is not just about including acupuncture, behavioral therapy, and mindfulness—treatments that we recommend to some patients—but isolating, testing, and treating each patient for every individual problem they have.

It is time to look at gluten differently and offer reliable science and guidance in navigating your way to a healthier and symptom-free life.

Part I exposes the many misconceptions surrounding gluten. The gluten-free diet works for many and is necessary for those with celiac disease. We now understand a great deal more about why it works, as well as the benefits and pitfalls of a gluten-free lifestyle. For others, the diet does not work—or works only for a short period of time—and understanding the reasons for that can help you reboot your health.

Where you get your medical and health information can determine whether you are being properly diagnosed, treated, and monitored on a diet that is not necessarily healthy. This includes taking a close look at your eating habits—you may be eliminating the wrong foods or your household may simply be too clean for your own immunological good. Most exclusion diets come at a price; you should know the precise value of what you are sacrificing.

We will examine the various temporary or expedient remedies that are being prescribed, including probiotics and supplements, to expose the underbelly, as it were, of this unregulated industry. We will explain the key tests that are used to analyze nutritional issues and symptoms that are often blamed on gluten but may mean something entirely different.

Having eliminated some of the myths, in **Part II** we will dive into the subterranean world of your gut, its many inhabitants, and how it communicates with your brain. Four of the hottest research topics today are the brain, the microbiome, inflammation, and the food we eat, gluten in particular. We have found new and intriguing connections between them.

We begin at the mouth, where food, drugs, supplements, tobacco, alcohol, "bugs" of all types, and anything else we knowingly or inadvertently swallow enter the body and travel through the digestive tract. But this is where the story gets interesting. For many, digestion is a torturous journey that creates gas, bloating, and pain in the gut. For others, food and other ingested substances create inflammation and multisystem disorders that radiate throughout the body.

Your gastrointestinal (GI) tract is in constant communication with your brain. Much of the story is actually narrated by our brains and the "second brain," the enteric nervous system in the gut. Thus, a dynamic interaction of multiple factors and "conversations" in the body determines not only your day-to-day but also your long-term health. In this section we will start to explore what happens when the gut talks to the brain and the brain answers back, and what each person can do to moderate this internal dialogue.

Part III examines the different elements that cause symptoms often attributed to gluten alone. This includes other portions of wheat and FODMAPs (fermentable oligosaccharides, disaccharides, monosaccharides, and polyols)—an acronym for the many dietary culprits in the carbohydrate family. Drugs, infections, and other illnesses also affect the gut-brain axis and disturb the microbiome. Many cause a "double hit"—the first infection or illness predisposing the body to a sensitivity to gluten. This will come as no surprise for anyone who has gotten turista or a traveler's infection; the bathroom journey often continues for months after they return. A double hit may even set the stage for schizophrenia.

This takes us to the role of inflammation and the so-called leaky gut, two largely misunderstood aspects of the body's defense system. They are blamed for many things they do not do—and implicated in others that we are just beginning to understand.

Part IV focuses on the specific conditions where gluten plays a part. Each section clarifies and explains the role and relation of diet, inflammation, antibodies, genes, germs, and gut-brain cross-talk, as well as the latest treatment options.

In Part V we look closely at the brain and separate pseudoscience from the important studies being conducted on serious and damaging conditions like autism and schizophrenia. We will look at the relation of gluten to "brain fog" and the potential long-term effects of the gluten-free diet on a person's mind and behavior. It is becoming increasingly clear that the constant need to "hold back" when eating—one of the most normal and usually pleasurable aspects of daily living—may create additional stress on both the brain and the body. Putting yourself on a restrictive diet—any diet—may have unintended consequences on the stress circuits in your brain.

For those committed to a truly gluten-free lifestyle, finding the right balance of nutritional foods is crucial, and Part VI will help to guide you there. This section contains the latest updates on nondietary therapies for celiac disease (the pharmaceutical products being developed to supplement or eliminate the need for a gluten-free diet), as well as further thoughts on what the science about gluten means for the future of our gut-brain health.

With a growing array of gluten-free products hitting the market almost monthly, it is important to know what is safe, what is hidden, and what are some of the nongluten ingredients in these products that are worse for the body than gluten. We will look at "food glue"—processed food doesn't grow that way—as well as the many myths that still surround a gluten-free diet.

Gluten is a piece in many medical puzzles but is the ultimate answer to only a few. We will help you determine if it is an answer to yours.

*Science, my lad, is made up of mistakes, but they are mistakes which
it is useful to make, because they lead little by little to the truth.*
—JULES VERNE, *JOURNEY TO THE CENTER OF THE EARTH*

*The scientific theory I like best is that the rings of Saturn
are composed entirely of lost airline luggage.*
—MARK RUSSELL

*Some people think that the truth can be hidden with a
little cover-up and decoration. But as time goes by, what
is true is revealed and what is fake fades away.*
—ISMAIL HANIYEH

PART I

Defining the Problem

It started with an avalanche of bad things happening. Kind of an achiness and gluey feelings in my joints all the time, and it just started to escalate. A mysterious fatigue where I just felt drugged.

The joint stuff was so bad I couldn't walk upstairs and couldn't roll over in bed without hurting. The final straw was when I developed vertigo, which got me to go to the doctor. I thought, *I'm too young for this to be going on.*

She did all these tests and scans, a neck X-ray, and everything was normal. She found "nothing wrong" with me. And yet I clearly was not functional.

Someone recommended removing things from my diet to see if it would help, and I started with wheat, dairy, sugar, and eggs. By the end of that first week I started to feel better and the vertigo went right away. It was literally like the tide going out. I was very disciplined and reintroduced each food, eggs first, then dairy, sugar, and wheat. When I reintroduced the wheat the back pain reappeared instantly.

(JILL, 50)*

I know a ton of people who don't eat gluten for a variety of things—or nothing.

(ANNABELLE, 33)

---

* In order to preserve patient confidentiality we have used first names or pseudonyms throughout.

The gluten hysteria is killing the credibility of people with celiac disease. Because people think it's a fad thing, that we're watching our weight or we think it is healthier, that we're choosing this way of life, and they're discounting the fact that it's a medical illness. You'd think we'd be going in a different direction. We've gone a few steps back.

(ILYSSA, 39)

What Is Your Source of Medical Information?

Science is a way of thinking much more than it is a body of knowledge.
—CARL SAGAN

I observe the physician with the same diligence as the disease.
—JOHN DONNE

I understand that I don't really know where I am on that gluten spectrum because I haven't had any tests. And the other stuff is treated like hocus-pocus. So individuals draw their own wacky conclusions. I'd really like to know what a scientist thinks about it and what I should do.

(JILL, 50)

There are many sources today for health information and many reasons individuals do not go to a doctor to get it. Many people will see a doctor only in order to resolve a physical ailment that has either disrupted their life, will not resolve itself in the over-the-counter (OTC) drug aisles of the pharmacy, or because their spouse/child/friend/sister, etc. insisted that "it's time to get to the bottom of this." In fact, many do not see a doctor until their symptoms have seriously affected their ability to work, travel, or sleep. And even then, some arrive with a list of answers before asking the physician what they think is the matter.

When was the last time you:

- Self-diagnosed from Internet information?
- Self-treated with OTC drugs and/or diet?
- Gave a doctor a diagnosis *before* you were examined?

Some people self-diagnose or seek alternative practitioners when medical tests fail to reveal a cause for ongoing symptoms and/or prescribed drugs fail to cure them. And many of them accept a food-related "diagnosis" as the solution to the problem. Given the current focus on foods as cause and cure, far too many roads lead to gluten. If you are looking to prove that gluten is the cause of your physical symptoms, you will undoubtedly find ammunition to justify this conclusion. As the scientist and mathematician John Lubbock noted: "What we see depends mainly on what we are looking for."

But if you type "gas, bloating, and fatigue" into your browser, you will find more than 90 other medical and psychiatric conditions on WebMD that cause the same symptoms. And your health depends on isolating, testing for, and treating the correct underlying condition.

My Doctor "Pooh-Poohs" Food Intolerances

When I don't eat gluten, I feel fine; when I do eat it, I don't. My doctor did all these tests and scans and X-rays, and everything was normal. She didn't say "it is in your head," but there was this long "Hmmmm. I don't have a diagnosis, but I think it's all about gluten."

(NANCY, 44)

Some physicians, aware of the popularity of the gluten-free diet and the susceptibility of people to dietary trends, dismiss nonceliac food intolerances as a legitimate cause for concern. These doctors may be dismissive of symptoms and therefore not interested in getting to the root of the problem, making diagnosis more difficult.

Doctors do not rely on Internet blogs, magazine articles, or website write-ups of scientific papers. They read and analyze the papers and base their diagnoses on peer-reviewed understanding of a condition. Medicine is a plastic science—studies change the understanding of diseases and their mechanisms regularly—so doctors treat conservatively rather than accepting what they may consider a diet that has no good "data" behind its efficacy. For this reason, some may believe that you are on a gluten-free diet for no real scientific reason.

Nevertheless, diagnosis is critical for social acceptance and accommodation—it confers legitimacy on a symptom or the patient. Thus, many people who feel marginalized by health care professionals turn to alternative practitioners to legitimatize their symptoms and solutions. This in turn undermines biomedical science and advocates self-diagnosis—an individual can avoid foods without a doctor's diagnosis. This can backfire if your problem has no relation to the food(s) you are eating. And if that is the case, you are postponing a proper diagnosis that might alleviate your symptoms.

Listening to the Media and the Masseuse

Many readers do not go beyond an article's headline or its opening paragraph; it is also difficult for laymen to critically assess statements coming from apparent voices of authority.
—JEROME GROOPMAN, M.D., *HOW DOCTORS THINK*

Health advice is readily available on the Internet, TV shows, and from nutritionists or unlicensed "dietitians," health gurus, masseuses, bloggers, newspapers, and magazines. While the advice from alternative sources can be helpful in some cases and generally ensures a sympathetic ear, it should not be a substitute for or confused with medical advice from your physician.

You Rely on Internet Advice

My patient arrived with a fistful of material from the Internet, a list of tests she wanted to confirm the diagnosis she'd come to of her problem, and possible drugs to treat it. I asked her why she bothered to consult with a doctor.

(DR. F)

There are many medical resources on the Internet, but it can be hard to understand and interpret research studies. PubMed Central, an archive of biomedical and life sciences journal literature at the U.S. National Institutes of Health's (NIH) National Library of Medicine, posts the abstracts of all research studies (essentially the summary of what the study set out to do and its results and conclusions). While some studies are free, obtaining full-text articles that contain a discussion section is often difficult without academic access and a subscription. This key section outlines all the limitations of the study (e.g., a very small group was tested, requiring confirmation in a larger study; participants dropped out because of symptoms; a drug or test caused serious side effects in a significant amount of people, etc.) that are crucial for assessing its meaning.

Magazine articles often trumpet a study, drug, or breakthrough that comes on the heels of another less-publicized study with opposing or lukewarm results.

Some Listserv sites distribute messages with Q&A sections to a specialized electronic mailing list. The advice on these sites ranges from practical travel and eating-out advice to testing analysis. The former is helpful; the latter is dangerous, as it comes mainly from patients.

Some people rely on the Internet more heavily because it is often financially difficult for them to see a doctor until a medical crisis sends them to the emergency room. Nevertheless, most major medical centers today have excellent websites based on the different specialties and conditions they treat. These specific sites offer reliable medical guidance and can help you determine if a doctor's visit is essential and help you to find appropriate resources.

Conflicting advice is found online, and many people read articles that agree with what they have already decided is the solution. Many are looking not for medical information but advice and treatments from the articles and "experts" that confirm their own prejudices on the subject.

The Internet offers everything from PubMed Central to preposterous—it is not a place to go for a diagnosis or treatment.

You "Test" Online

Alternative tests for various food intolerances are available online. While the less said about them the better—you are paying a great deal of money for something that is scientifically meaningless—the reasons behind this statement deserve some explanation.

A biological marker for gluten sensitivity does not currently exist, although researchers are working to find one. (See chapter 18, "Gluten Sensitivity.") Despite that fact, fecal (stool) tests for this condition are available online along with other fecal tests for various food intolerances and allergies. The same "lab" also advertises a DNA genetic test for nonceliac gluten sensitivity (NCGS) even though no specific genes have been isolated for the condition.

Additionally, the markers they claim will determine the "diagnosis" (IgG antigliadin antibodies) are neither sensitive nor specific enough to diagnose either celiac disease or gluten sensitivity. (See chapter 6, "A Word on Testing.") It has been shown that 20 percent of non-gluten-sensitive individuals also have elevated levels of these antibodies for no apparent reason, which puts any "diagnosis" by these tests in serious doubt.

The danger of getting your medical information and diagnosis from what amounts to a self-test is that your problem may not be gluten sensitivity and you fail to get a proper medical evaluation, thereby missing a serious illness that then goes untreated and may progress.

You Do It "Naturally" with Alternative Sources

Inundated by headlines and articles exposing the dangers in our food supply, the side effects of drugs, the rise in hospital-borne infections, bacterial resistance to antibiotics, and many other environmental dangers, many patients want a more "natural" approach to health care. Others feel that they understand their bodies better than their doctors. While there may be some truth in this thinking, it can also border on the delusional. (See chapter 3, "Picky Eaters.")

Many people find their thinking about food and fatigue issues is more simpatico with that of a chiropractor, trainer, nutritionist, or acupuncturist and follow their dietary and supplement advice. Some of these practitioners push products that they claim will cure gastrointestinal issues, cleanse the body, and enhance your health, but are usually the modern version of snake oil—a quick quack remedy or panacea. The majority of these products will do little more than help your wallet lose weight, and some of them can be truly dangerous. (See chapter 5, "Supplements and Probiotics.") This can make patients fearful or unwilling to tell their doctors about the supplements, herbs, and potions they take in addition to prescription medications. The doctor is then unable to unravel a drug/supplement interaction that could be lethal and would be immediately apparent if the patient had come clean.

Doing it "naturally" or on your own can compound issues, especially when there are major problems or psychological issues.

Why Individuals Don't Go to Doctors

Whenever I read anything, it says, "Consult your doctor before doing any exercise." Does anybody do that? I kind of think my doctor has people coming in with serious problems. I don't think I should be calling him and saying, "Hi, this is Rita, I'm thinking of bending at the waist."

—RITA RUDNER

There are various reasons people do not rely on doctors for medical advice and treatment, but food and lifestyle issues seem to raise a red flag on both sides of the desk. Many with unresolved symptoms assume the doctor trivializes them as nonserious and therefore they avoid the discussion. Others state that they think the doctor views a gluten-free diet as a lifestyle rather than a health decision. And if going gluten-free is not to treat celiac disease, a wheat allergy, or another diagnosed condition but gives you a better quality of life, you both may be right.

My Doctor Doesn't Listen/Have Time

My doctor said, "You have celiac disease. Go on a gluten-free diet and I'll see you in six months." That's when we got really frustrated and really lost. My doctor sent me home without any guidance.

(ARLENE, 18)

Admittedly, not every doctor is a talented listener. Understanding the experience of illness comes with practice, and some physicians need to be reminded that the antibodies on the lab sheet are attached to a person. But there are two sides to this dialogue, and patients often fashion their narratives to give the doctor what they think the doctor wants to hear. The result can be unsatisfactory for both parties.

Allergies and food intolerances—along with celiac disease and other autoimmune diseases—have mushroomed in the past decade for reasons that are still being actively researched. Many physicians are therefore still examining the dietary and potential microbiotic aspects of their specialties, so you should request a professional referral for dietary counseling if your diagnosis requires a restricted diet.

Food restriction is currently the only treatment for those with celiac disease and food allergies, and a major component of others, such as diabetes and kidney stones. Trained and registered dietitians have the time to explore the nuances of these various diets, and you should turn to them for expert advice after—not before—diagnosis.

You Got Off on the Wrong Floor

*Where you stand depends on where you sit: your specialty
can affect, even determine, your position.*
—JEROME GROOPMAN, M.D., *HOW DOCTORS THINK*

Many people look to alternative sources for a diagnosis because they feel that their doctor "sees me only as someone with irritable bowel syndrome." Diagnoses stick until it can be proven that you have something else—and negative test results often leave people categorized and displeased with the answer. Patients with GI symptoms usually have GI issues; those with neurological symptoms usually have neurological issues. Doctors are taught in medical school that "the common occurs commonly." But frequently GI issues can cause neurological symptoms, as is seen in celiac disease and other malabsorption conditions that cause vitamin and mineral deficiencies leading to *ataxia** (lack of coordination) and other gut-brain reactions.

If you need a raincoat, you won't find it in the shoe department. It is often necessary to run different tests or seek out a different specialist who is willing to change his/her position on an issue.

Financial Issues

The insurance and financial landscape of medicine is a reason cited by some people in the U.S. to explain their avoidance of medical care. If you continue to have unresolved symptoms and are self-diagnosing and self-treating without the benefit of medical testing, you should seek out a clinic or practice that will accommodate your needs, before an underlying condition sends you to the emergency room.

---

* Throughout the book we italicize less-familiar words and terms when they first appear and provide a more complete definition in the glossary at the back of the book.

Where you get your medical information will ultimately determine your long-term health.

Ask yourself if you are seeking alternative sources of medical information mainly to justify a gluten-free diet as the answer for ongoing symptoms. As 19th-century French physiologist Claude Bernard said, "It is what we think we know already that often prevents us from learning."

2

Does a Gluten-Free Diet Work for You?

You have to decide that food is no longer the focus of your life.

(DINA, 28)

It's harming people with celiac disease because people are choosing the "diet of the month," and it's really impacting the people who medically are on a restricted diet.

(JEAN, 37)

Are You a PWAG?

PWAGs (pronounced *pee-wags*) stands for people who avoid wheat and gluten. It is a term coined by a group of gastroenterologists to encompass the huge numbers of patients they have been seeing who go on a gluten-free diet because of what they describe as an intolerance to wheat products in the absence of celiac disease.

Many of these patients have a higher prevalence of the genes associated with celiac disease (the HLA-DQ typing). And one study showed that PWAGs had a higher number of medical diagnoses for other food intolerances and *small intestine bacterial overgrowth (SIBO)*.

If you are a PWAG, there are many reasons you made this decision—disease treatment, symptoms relief, perception of a healthier way to be, recommended by a health care professional, etc. And an equal variation in its success.

First and Foremost—What Is Gluten?

Gluten is the general term used to describe the storage protein of wheat. Wheat is approximately 10 to 15 percent protein—the remainder is starch. Gluten is what remains after the starch granules are washed from wheat flour. The gluten fraction that is most studied in celiac disease is *gliadin*, but there are other proteins that chemically resemble *gliadin* in rye (secalins) and barley (hordeins). These proteins are not strictly glutens, but are generally included in the term. There are other proteins in wheat (see chapter 11, "Gluten and Nongluten Grains") that may also be problematic for PWAGs and are part of the complex reason why the diet works for some, only partially for others, or not at all.

Why a Gluten-Free Diet Works

You have celiac disease and the diet fixes the inflamed intestine.

A gluten-free diet is a lifesaver for those with celiac disease and is a proven medical treatment. If followed carefully, it resolves symptoms, rebuilds nutritional stores depleted by a damaged intestinal lining, and, in children, rebuilds bone loss caused by malabsorption of calcium. (See chapter 17, "Celiac Disease.")

You have nonceliac gluten sensitivity (NCGS) and the diet relieves symptoms (neurological, skin, gastrointestinal).

Many individuals who feel or have been told that they have NCGS—again, there are currently no diagnostic tests for this condition—find relief with gluten withdrawal for neurological disorders, skin rashes, and GI symptoms such as gas and bloating. (See chapter 18, "Gluten Sensitivity.")

You have irritable bowel syndrome (IBS), and elimination diets have resolved some or all of the gas, bloating, and pain.

IBS may be due to a sensitivity to a food that most tolerate without problems. It is a diagnosis of exclusion—other tests having proven negative—and dietary restriction can be successful, often only partially, for those patients with carbohydrate intolerances. (See chapter 12, "Carbohydrates and FODMAPs," and chapter 19, "Irritable Bowel Syndrome.")

You just think it works so it does.

A placebo is not only the archetypal sugar pill but anything that impacts a patient's expectations.

Why a Gluten-Free Diet Does Not Work

The main reason a gluten-free diet does not work is that gluten is not the issue and/or you may be missing treatment for another disease.

This may include:

- SIBO
- Fructose intolerance
- Lactose intolerance
- Other food intolerances
- Microscopic colitis
- Gastroparesis (a condition where the stomach cannot empty properly)
- Pelvic floor dysfunction (weak muscles in the pelvic floor, often caused by childbirth)
- A problem related to a medication you are taking

After a thorough medical evaluation, we find that many PWAGs have a variety of conditions and may, in fact, be able to eat gluten again, symptom free, with proper diagnosis and treatment.

You may be on a gluten-free diet but other types of carbohydrates, e.g., fructose, are the problem. (See chapter 12, "Carbohydrates and FODMAPs.")

You're under the impression that the diet is a cure-all for many health-related ailments.

A survey by *Consumer Reports* showed that 63 percent of North Americans think that a gluten-free diet improves physical or mental health, and 33 percent buy gluten-free products because they believe these foods will improve digestion and gastrointestinal function. Unless you have celiac disease or a specific carbohydrate intolerance, a gluten-free diet will not work for either of these issues.

The diet does not work to lower cholesterol or strengthen your immune system, even though many people believe it does.

The diet is disrupting your intestinal flora—the microbiome— and causing symptoms.

Restrictive diets—gluten-free, low-FODMAP—have been shown to reduce the richness and diversity of our intestinal microbiota, which in turn may cause persistent symptoms in patients with celiac disease and possibly other conditions. While it is unclear exactly what this disruption means or the long-term effects, it is generally believed that a diverse microbiome is healthier. While there is no one "healthy" microbiome, the studies on this should be watched. (For more, see chapter 9, "The Microbiome.")

People should make every effort to diversify their diets. This may be particularly important as people age. Aging is known to be associated with a reduced diversity of the gut microbiome, and this may lead to a compromised intestinal barrier and increased susceptibility to infectious diseases and infections.

If a disrupted microbiome is a side effect of a gluten-free diet, these consequences should be considered before you embark on a gluten-free regimen unless you have celiac disease.

Will It Work in Other Ways?

Can I lose weight on a gluten-free diet?

Some go on a gluten-free diet to lose weight. This works if you exclude but do not replace wheat as the main carbohydrate. In animal studies a gluten-free diet prevented the development of obesity and metabolic disorders. BUT, while gluten was eliminated from the diet, the mice were not fed replacements with gluten-free products. The no–white food or Atkins diet (no bread, pasta, potatoes, rice, cake, or cookies) will usually ensure weight loss but can be nutritionally inadequate if enough fruit and vegetables are not substituted for those carbohydrates. It is also hard to sustain.

Will I have more energy?

Unfortunately, if you do not have celiac disease, a gluten-free diet is not likely to make you the Energizer Bunny. Although many people insist that they feel logy or tired after eating gluten, there is little scientific evidence to support this. Postprandial fatigue (which occurs after eating) is common, especially after a large meal, when various hormones are released to aid digestion. These hormones act on the brain when released in the gut and cause the fatigue many report.

Will I become a world-class athlete—or will thinking so make it better?

The use of a gluten-free diet by famous people has enhanced its appeal. Publicized by Hollywood stars, it has also been endorsed by several high-profile athletes. The reasons behind this speak to our infatuations with celebrities and fad diets, and wanting to believe something enough to think it works—the placebo effect.[*]

An Australian study of nonceliac athletes, including eighteen world and/or Olympic medalists who followed a gluten-free diet 50 to 100 percent of the time, reported that self-diagnosed gluten sensitivity was the primary reason for adopting the diet. The leading sources of information on the gluten-free diet were online, a trainer/coach, and other athletes. Neither the diagnosis nor treatment was based on medical rationale, merely the perception that removing gluten provided "health benefits" and an "ergogenic edge."

If you do not have chronic symptoms that require medical treatment, the gluten-free diet can be both placebo and minefield. We advise staying tuned to your local news for updates—the latest dietary trend may be announced on *Entertainment Tonight*.

If you are looking for more realistic scientific advice, the following chapters will explore what taking gluten and other foods out of your diet will really do to and for your body.

---

[*] Or the "nocebo" effect, where believing something will harm you actually causes an adverse reaction to it.

3

Picky Eaters—Orthorexia and the Hygiene Hypothesis

Water surges, only to overflow.
—CHINESE PROVERB

Things turn into their opposites when they reach their extremes. And "healthy" eating is moving in that direction.

There are good reasons that we have food on our minds. According to the U.S. Centers for Disease Control and Prevention (CDC), half of all Americans have a chronic disease or condition such as high blood pressure, heart disease, or type 2 diabetes and have been instructed to think about fat, sugar, and/or salt. More than 9 percent have diabetes and must monitor their sugar/glucose intake multiple times every day. At least 35 percent of Americans are obese and cycle through different diets, gaining and losing weight every year. About 1 percent has celiac disease and avoids gluten. Up to 15 million people in the U.S. have a food allergy, estimated to affect 1 in every 13 children under the age of 18. A study by the World Health Organization reported that noncommunicable diseases were responsible for 86 percent of all deaths and 77 percent of the disease burden in the European Region and noted that this primarily included conditions caused by high blood pressure and cardiovascular diseases. Three of the priority interventions recommended were dietary.

Unfortunately, the National Eating Disorders Association notes that 20 million women and 10 million men suffered from a clinically significant eating disorder at some point in their life, including anorexia nervosa, bulimia, binge eating, or an eating disorder not otherwise specified. In the UK, a National Health Service (NHS) study estimated that more than 725,000 people are affected by an eating disorder and that eating disorders can affect people of any age.

The current obsession with food is not surprising; mankind has been on some kind of restricted diet—by need or choice—since the beginning of time (see Appendix A), but for some it has taken a turn into the obsessively unhealthy.

Orthorexia Nervosa—Healthy Eating as a Disease

Food is an important part of a balanced diet.
—FRAN LEBOWITZ

I don't like anything "lite"—that's not my thing. I have one friend who goes to a chiropractor who tests you, and they take one thing after another out of your diet. He evaluates what you eat and decides what foods your body is not tolerating. She's currently living on kale.

(ILYSSA, 39)

The focus of the press and social media on "healthy eating" as the source of, or cure for, disease has taken hold to the point of creating a new condition termed *orthorexia nervosa*. Individuals eliminate one healthy food after another (gluten, corn, soy, meat, dairy, all fats, carbohydrates, etc.) in the belief that these foods are "unhealthy"—until they are barely receiving adequate nourishment. It can reach the point of anemia, bone loss, vitamin depletion, and malnutrition.

The condition is not as yet recognized in the *DSM-V* (the *Diagnostic and Statistical Manual of Mental Disorders,* used professionally to diagnose psychiatric disorders) but is being seen by many doctors evaluating patients for symptoms related to nutritional deficiencies.

The term *orthorexia* was coined by Dr. Steven Bratman from the Greek *ortho* (correct or proper) and *orexis* (hunger or appetite). Unlike in anorexia, those with orthorexia focus on the *quality* rather than the *quantity* of food eaten. They start removing foods because they do not feel well, and when they do not feel better, they remove more and more until they are on an overly restricted and generally unhealthy diet.

Are You Orthorexic?

- Have you eliminated entire food groups from your diet? (Gluten, dairy, corn, and soy are the usual suspects as well as red meat, carbohydrates, etc.)
- Three or more food groups?
- Do you constantly worry about which foods may be unhealthy?
- Do you feel guilty when you eat food you consider unsafe?
- Do you have problems finding healthy foods?
- Do you have ritualized eating patterns?
- Are you anxious when eating out or traveling?
- Have you started avoiding lunches, dinner dates, and catered parties?
- Do you lecture your friends and family about unhealthy eating?
- Do you read medical journal articles about digestion, carbohydrates, protein, etc.?
- Do you challenge others who disagree with your food choices?

- Do you wish that you could just eat and not worry about the quality of foods?
- Do you have symptoms that do not fit any medical diagnostic category for which you blame gluten, dairy, or a specific food?

Orthorexia affects a small percentage of individuals, but is yet another food-related disorder that has evolved from the increased focus on food as cause and/or cure for symptoms and disease.

The Hygiene Hypothesis—Are We Too Clean for Our Own Immunological Good?

My daughter-in-law sterilizes everything that goes into my grandson's mouth. I raised four children on the 10-second rule—if it's been on the floor for less than 10 seconds, pick it up and eat it—and not one had an allergy or food issue. Now we're boiling the baby's fork and spoon after it comes out of the dishwasher, and every other person's child is allergic to peanuts or dairy or gluten. Something's wacky here.

(GERI, 64)

The diagnosis of allergies and autoimmune diseases has risen dramatically in the last few decades. While there are many underlying and complex mechanisms at work, a great deal of scientific interest is being focused on the "hygiene hypothesis." This states that childhood exposure to germs and certain infections helps the immune system develop normally, and that excessive cleanliness interrupts this process.

In other words, the young child's environment can be too clean to effectively challenge a maturing immune system. Frequent and repeated exposure to a variety of *microbial antigens* and infections may lead to a more robust, i.e., healthier immune system.

While it is well documented that avoiding germs helps prevent the spread of infections, the hygiene hypothesis suggests that we have taken this too far. And with the advent of antibiotics and the great public health efforts of the last century, the immune system is no longer required to fight germs as actively as in the past.

Scientists based this hypothesis in part on the observation that, before birth, the fetal immune system's "default setting" is suppressed to prevent it from rejecting the mother's tissue. This is necessary before birth—when the mother is providing the fetus with her own antibodies. After birth the child's own immune system must take over and learn how to fend for itself. But the extremely clean household environments often found in the developed world do not provide the necessary exposure to germs required to "educate" the immune system so that it can learn to launch its defense responses to infectious organisms.

A critical part of this evolution is orchestrated by a child's developing microbiome, and a lack of diversity—reduced by exposure to fewer germs and infections—derails the period of immune growth after birth.

The hygiene hypothesis has been implicated in the growing number of people with allergies, autism, and autoimmune diseases.

MacDonald's Farm Had the Right Idea?

Since the hypothesis was first proposed by epidemiologist Dr. David Strachan in 1989, several studies have revealed a reduction in the sensitivity to allergens and atopic (skin) disease in children exposed to farm environments, those who have animals in their homes, and in those who have attended day care at an early age and were exposed to other children's infections.

Several lessons have come from studies comparing populations in Russian Karelia and neighboring Finland. These two populations live in completely different socioeconomic circumstances—they have one of the largest socioeconomic discrepancies in the world—yet share similar diets and genetic backgrounds.

The researchers determined that the children in Karelia are exposed to a large variety of different microbial infections that are significantly less frequent in Finnish children. Starting in 1999, numerous studies on autoimmune and allergic diseases show an incidence of type 1 diabetes that is six times lower in Russian Karelia. The incidence of celiac disease is 1 in 496 in Karelia and 1 in 107 in Finland using identical criteria. These studies appear to indicate that environmental factors play a role in our immune reaction to microbes and in the development of allergies and autoimmune conditions. While all of the factors initiating these conditions have not been identified, the hygiene hypothesis offers an intriguing approach.

The mechanisms by which microbes can reduce the development of autoimmune disease are not well understood. They are only part of a larger autoimmune and allergic response that is also affected by your genetic makeup, and a variety of factors that occur over a person's lifetime. It cannot be considered the sole determinant of a disease.

Before people start feeding their children from the floor or allowing them to share the dog's bowl, it should be stressed that many researchers feel that the hygiene hypothesis is far too simplistic an approach to understanding the causes of celiac disease or any other autoimmune disease.

This hypothesis does focus attention on the impact of microbes on disease, hopefully without discouraging good hygiene practices.

BOTH ORTHOREXIA AND the hygiene hypothesis are extreme examples, yet they illustrate what can happen when individuals become mesmerized by the message, and the human body is deprived of the many forms of nourishment it requires to develop, grow, and flourish. Both advanced in the name of "health."

What we deprive our body of is every bit as important as what we feed it.

4

Pitfalls and Perils of a Gluten-Free Diet

Sooner or later everyone sits down to a banquet of consequences.
—R. L. STEVENSON

A gluten-free diet gives with one hand and takes away with the other. For individuals with celiac disease, it truly is a lifesaver yet requires constant vigilance and restrictions. Others find it gives them relief from symptoms like gas and bloating while taking many essential nutrients from their diets. The "giving hand" can also contain heavy metals, toxins, and excess fat and sugar. The "taking hand" dips into pocketbooks for more costly foods. The scale can get very unbalanced if individuals are not aware of the health risks in a gluten-free diet that are often hidden behind the hype surrounding it.

Studies on the real long-term effects of a gluten-free diet on the body and the brain are being published with increasing regularity since the awareness of celiac disease and popularity of the diet in the general public began about a decade ago. While many of the studies are on celiac disease patients who must follow a strict gluten-free diet, research has exposed some troubling issues that affect everyone following the diet.

Mostly we are doing it because we realized how good we can feel and believe it is healthy for us.

(ARIELLE, 33)

A gluten-free diet is many things to many people, but for most it is far from healthy.

Healthy or Hazardous?

Nutrition

Going "gluten-free" may cure symptoms for some, and is a necessity for those with celiac disease, but eliminating gluten from your diet also removes much of the fiber and some essential vitamins and minerals from your food supply.

Wheat, rye, and barley are flavorful, vitamin- and fiber-filled grains. Ironically, manufacturers also regularly fortify wheat flours as well as the cereals, breads, and other processed products made from them with the vitamins and minerals that might have been removed during processing. Conversely, gluten-free foods, with a few exceptions, have not caught up with this fortification. Some, like quinoa, may not need this as much as rice flour.

The breads, cereals, cookies, cakes, and snacks with gluten-free grains also put people at risk for potential problems with excess fat, sugar, and salt. These ingredients are used to bind gluten-free products—gluten is the "glue" that holds breads and cakes together—and to make them as tasty as their wheat-filled counterparts.

People with celiac disease who embark on a gluten-free diet without the help of a nutritionist can easily develop vitamin and mineral deficiencies, especially iron and the B vitamins. Calcium can also be deficient if dairy is restricted. This is a double problem because many start the diet already suffering from malabsorption due to the damage to their small intestine. Missing a favorite sweet or breaded dish, they often make poor food choices to satisfy a craving.

Lost fiber and nutrients need to be replaced with fresh fruits, nuts, beans, vegetables, and other gluten-free grains (e.g., quinoa, millet, buckwheat, sorghum) to maintain a "nutritional" diet. If you are going to take gluten out, put its nutritional value back in. (For more, see chapter 31, "Eating Healthy.")

Heavy Metal (Not of the Musical Variety)

Rice, a common substitute in a gluten-free diet, may contain high levels of arsenic as well as cadmium and mercury. Other heavy metals (e.g., tin, lead, and mercury) have also been found both in gluten-free food and flours and the people ingesting them.

While the raised levels do not approach toxic levels, there should be a warning. A greater number of patients with celiac disease develop neurological symptoms over the ensuing years after starting a gluten-free diet. While this has been attributed to the development of a new autoimmune disease, the recent concern about the occurrence of metals such as lead, mercury, and arsenic in people on a gluten-free diet may in fact be a manifestation of heavy metal toxicity.

Arsenic with Your Rice?

Arsenic occurs naturally in the environment and is also released into soil and water by fertilizers and pesticides as well as manufacturing practices. It is absorbed into anything growing in these environments—in particular, rice absorbs arsenic more readily than many other plants. The Environmental Protection Agency (EPA) published a "hazard summary" about arsenic in 2012 stating that "food is the major source of exposure" for most people and that chronic exposure can result in GI effects as well as central and peripheral nervous system disorders and certain cancers. Studies suggest that it may also affect a baby's immune system when ingested by a mother during pregnancy.

The Food and Drug Administration (FDA) has not released a finished assessment of the potential health risks associated with arsenic in rice and other foods made from rice, but *Consumer Reports* and other studies urge caution.

Consumer Reports tested several different rices from growing regions around the world and concluded that organic rice is no different from conventionally grown rice—they both take up arsenic in the same manner from soil and water. Brown rice often has the highest levels because metallic elements accumulate in the husk and bran, which are milled off when rice is processed. Nevertheless, brown rice still contains more nutrients and is more fibrous.

It is possible to reduce the risk of arsenic in cooked rice by rinsing the raw rice before cooking, and by using excess water during the cooking process and throwing it out before serving; this sacrifices some nutritional value but can reduce the arsenic content by almost a third.

Almost everything that's gluten-free has some rice in it. Suzanne Simpson, R.D., of the Celiac Disease Center at Columbia University cautions patients: "Rice doesn't have a lot of nutritional value. It doesn't have a lot of fiber or protein; it is basically just carbs. Most of the [gluten-free] breads, pasta, tortillas, cookies, and flour mixes contain rice. And people eat rice on top of it." Children who are on a gluten-free diet that also contains rice pasta, cookie, and bread products as well as cooked rice should be monitored to lessen arsenic exposure.

She recommends that people do not use rice pasta and minimize their rice intake for variety as well. We also advise people on a gluten-free diet to see a dietitian regularly to ensure that the diet is diverse and not simply various versions of rice. (See Appendix C, "Arsenic and Mercury Guidelines.")

Corn Fungi

The other grain staple of a gluten-free diet is corn. A recent study comparing the gluten-free diet of people with celiac disease versus those on a regular diet found a mycotoxin (a chemical produced by fungi/mold that is harmful to humans and domestic animals) in a number of corn products. The levels of this particular mycotoxin—a fumonisin associated with nervous-system and cancer-causing damage in animals—were high, raising concern regarding the long-term safety of various corn-based products.

The contamination of corn products with fumonisins has also been reported in other European studies, suggesting the potential of toxicity for anyone on a gluten-free diet ingesting a fair amount of corn-based products. While little is known about the fumonisin in the American diet, it is an area for further research and emphasizes the need to diversify the diet!

Mercury and Other Metals

Mercury is a naturally occurring heavy metal that appears to be increasing/accumulating in the food chain because of its use in medications, dental amalgams, thermometers, blood pressure machines, batteries, and fluorescent lightbulbs, and its presence in the fish we eat. Mercury can damage the nervous system, kidney, and lungs and remains in the body for a long time, where it affects inflammation and the immune system.

A recent study showed a fourfold increase in mercury blood levels of celiac disease patients following a gluten-free diet. No differences were found in their fish intake or number of amalgam fillings—both sources of mercury found to increase the amount of this metal in the body—but other dietary sources were not examined. Another study found elevated blood levels of mercury, lead, and cadmium and urinary levels of tin and arsenic in people eating a gluten-free diet, some with and some without celiac disease.

The reason for the increased levels in these people is unclear—whether it is food related, altered absorption, or response to mercury in these people. There might also be a genetic tendency in these people to accumulate it or to be more susceptible to specific toxic effects.

Additional studies to determine what is causing the increase in heavy metals in people following a gluten-free diet are needed. It is a potential pitfall that cannot be ignored.

Gluten Weighing In

The weight-loss potential of a gluten-free diet seems to be one of its biggest attractions for some people. Numerous Hollywood names attest to its effectiveness. If you cut out all bread, pasta, cake, cookies, and snacks and do not replace them with gluten-free alternatives, you will probably lose weight. It's called the no–white food, no-carb, gluten-free diet.

But many people following a gluten-free diet are surprised when they find themselves gaining weight from the many fat-, sugar-, and sodium-filled gluten-free products they are now eating to replace what has been removed. People with a double diagnosis of diabetes and celiac disease who must count carbohydrates are initially surprised to see that the gluten-free substitute is often much higher in carbs.

> I was eating everything—and constantly—and lost 25 pounds in the year before I was diagnosed (with celiac disease). Once I went on a gluten-free diet, I ate the same amount and gained 30 pounds in about seven months. I went from sick and skinny to healthy and chubby. The pasta and bread and cakes were gluten-free and didn't go right through me, so I realized I had to retrain and restrain myself.
>
> (SHEILA, 46)

People with celiac disease also often gain weight on a gluten-free diet because their intestine is healing and they are now able to digest food properly. Depending on how you define "going gluten-free," you may actually find that one of the things it "gives" is added pounds.

No Shelf Life Means More Money

The costs involved in buying shelf space from the retailer are prohibitive for the smaller manufacturer. It is one of the reasons why you see mainly larger national brands in your local stores. Also, the range and types of ingredients we use are more costly, and gluten-

> free products fit in the "natural" and "organic" world, where retail-
> ers often charge a premium over regular products. Many items
> are also made by smaller manufacturers who don't have the same
> big-company processing efficiency. These are some of the reasons
> gluten-free food is costlier.
>
> —GEORGE CHOOKAZIAN, FOODS BY GEORGE

Gluten-free products are generally much more expensive and less widely available than their gluten counterparts. There are a number of reasons that manufacturers give for this.

Ingredients as well as facilities have to be certified and adhere to specific labeling regulations and testing, which incurs costs. Ingredients must also be grown and milled contamination-free and are often purchased in smaller batches than those used by larger manufacturers, again adding expenses. Many breads, cakes, and muffins are frozen to preserve their freshness. They have a shorter shelf life than preservative-filled products, and spoilage adds to their cost.

Some manufacturers have started lowering prices as competition in the market increases, but gluten-free products can still add to a family's grocery bill.

You Have Isolated the Wrong Issue

One of the biggest dangers of going on a gluten-free diet before properly isolating and testing for what is causing symptoms is postponing and/or missing a correct diagnosis. Numerous other serious medical conditions—including microscopic colitis, SIBO, inflammatory bowel disease (IBD), and irritable bowel syndrome (IBS)—often present with the same symptoms as food-induced dyspepsia or other GI complaints. Gas, bloating, pain, diarrhea, and constipation can be distress signals for almost any and every GI disorder and disease. And neuropathies, headache, and fatigue can signal a number of underlying autoimmune and neurological diseases.

Many people mistakenly believe that their symptoms can be treated and cured through food elimination. By the time you finally get to a doctor, the gluten-free diet may have intensified another condition and taken away your health.

You May Be Eating Gluten Anyway

The biggest hurdles? Contamination. If I had to sum it up, I'm very comfortable with the lifestyle, very comfortable feeding my family, the options are enormous, but I never sit down at a dinner and say, "This is perfectly right." The kids want pizza and pasta. But when they have gluten-free pasta on the menu I still worry that they don't know how to prepare it safely. I still struggle with it.

(ILYSSA, 39)

One pitfall in a gluten-free diet is trying to adhere to it when gluten is a hidden ingredient in or on your food. This may be due to contamination or confusion about gluten-free labeling and regulations or actual false labeling.

Cross-contamination and a lack of awareness in restaurants accounts for most of the "I got glutened" comments from people trying to follow a gluten-free diet. For preparing gluten-free meals, restaurant kitchens often use fryers or pasta water in which dishes that are breaded or contain gluten have been cooked. The cross-contamination that occurs in manufacturing also usually relates to shared equipment, confusion about barley and malt—which contain gluten but not from wheat, which is required to be listed as an allergen on labels—or gluten that finds its way from crops that share fields and storage facilities with non-gluten grains.

Testing can be spotty. Several groups offer "gluten-free certification," but they are not all using the same ELISA (enzyme-linked immunosorbent assay) tests to ascertain gluten content. It is also physically impossible to test every batch of a cereal or packaged product to ensure that it contains less than 20 parts per million, the standard set by the FDA for all foods with a "gluten-free" label.

Reading labels and talking to food servers is crucial to avoiding hidden ingredients and cross-contamination. Doing so is a source of stress and disruption for many people.

> We were in a restaurant with a gluten-free menu, so I probably didn't ask enough questions. But my daughter ate the salad and what looked like a plain chicken breast, and within 20 minutes she was vomiting all over the tablecloth. I knew she'd gotten gluten no matter what they told me.
>
> (CISSY, 42)

> Whenever we go away I go right to the head of food services in every hotel. I don't bombard them but ask how they can help me and how I can help them. So they have the knowledge for the next person who comes with celiac disease. We get amazing dedication and great service.
>
> (ILYSSA, 39)

Less Microbiotic Diversity

Any restrictive diet reduces the diversity of the microbiota in the gastrointestinal tract, a potentially unhealthy change. While there is no one healthy microbiome, a gluten-free diet removes foods that the intestinal microbiota dine on. Studies show that the FODMAP diet may not be a healthy one to maintain for that reason, and patients are cautioned about the consequences of remaining on it for a long period of time. (See chapter 5, "Supplements and Probiotics.")

The Bottom Line

A gluten-free diet is lifesaving for people with celiac disease. It reduces symptoms for many with NCGS—people who have tested negative for celiac disease but who have similar symptoms—and IBS. But the long-term harm of the diet for people who do not really need it is still unknown.

What we do know is that a gluten-free diet is:

- low in fiber
- low in iron
- low in B vitamins
- high in sugar and fat
- associated with elevated levels of heavy metals in the body
- a risk for increased sensitivity to gluten
- potentially bad for your microbiome

Be advised that when embarking on a gluten-free diet you are potentially sitting down to a banquet of consequences. If you are thinking of replacing what is lost in a gluten-free diet with supplements and probiotics, read the °next chapter carefully.

5

Supplements and Probiotics

I had watched a TV show with [a well-known doctor] when he talked about a supplement—garcinia cambogia—for weight loss. The doctor had a very good reputation, and he seemed to think it was a good thing. A number of my friends love the show, and it's impressive, very persuasive. I thought it seemed safe, and I took that for about a month. I didn't feel any different, and I didn't lose any weight but happened to see my doctor right before we were going on a trip to Mexico. The doctor called me over the weekend when he got my blood tests back and told me that I had hepatitis.

I thought, *What!?* It was unbelievable! Garcinia cambogia was so popular and so heavily advertised, and I thought that it didn't seem like anything risky. My advice to someone taking something recommended on TV—don't trust them or take anything without talking to your doctor first. Vitamins and supplements are an unregulated industry. This could have killed me and severely damaged my liver. I seem to have recovered completely but have to be checked regularly. I thought, *It's just a plant*—I guess there's nothing more lethal than nature.

(CAROL, 56)

Carol had acute drug-induced hepatitis that can be progressive and result in liver failure and even death. Luckily hers resolved because it was caught in time. She had a follow-up appointment at the Center early in the development of the disease, and a medical history showed that she had recently started taking garcinia cambogia for weight loss. She stopped taking the drug after blood tests pinpointed the problem. The literature prominently lists hepatotoxicity (liver toxicity) as a side effect of garcinia cambogia—weight loss is not.

Hepatitis does not cause symptoms early in the disease, just biochemical evidence of acute hepatitis in the form of elevated liver enzymes. Later, symptoms of liver failure develop, including nausea, vomiting, anorexia, confusion, and coma. Drug-induced liver failure may result in death if not caught early. Carol soon learned what "just a plant" meant—and that "natural" does not mean "harmless."

Half of all Americans take some type of herbal remedy, and more than $28 billion a year is spent on various vitamins, minerals, herbal preparations, and probiotics. This number is about $104 billion globally. While visits to medical professionals have remained steady over the past decade, consultations with alternative medical practitioners and health gurus have increased dramatically—along with the use of supplements.

A tsunami of herbs, minerals, vitamins, and probiotics fill the shelves in drugstores, natural food stores, and supermarkets. They are heavily advertised not just as dietary supplements but as good for your health and claim to treat a wide spectrum of conditions from prostate problems and depression to sexual dysfunction, anxiety, insomnia, thinning hair, weight loss, and more. They are also promoted as a pharmaceutical aid for diarrhea, gas, and bacteria lost through antibiotic use, vaginal yeast infections, oncoming colds and flu, and pain. Many believe that they are safer than prescription drugs whose adverse effects are stated in accompanying literature.

> I read the warning label on the [drug] my doctor prescribed—it was longer than my college thesis. Looked as if it would probably cure me if it didn't kill me first. The labels on my supplements have no [listed] side effects of note.
>
> (SHARON, 65)

They've been using these as medical cures in China for centuries.

(ANGELA, 33)

The fact that they have been used for thousands of years in the East may be the only justifiable claim many supplements can make. Although there is little scientific evidence to support the medical claims made in the popular media about the effectiveness of supplements, most people consider them "natural" and basically safe. But several recent and scientifically rigorous studies have proved that there are some very dangerous trends in this unregulated industry, and some supplements may have life-threatening consequences. A recent study in the *New England Journal of Medicine* showed that approximately 23,000 emergency room visits each year—between the years 2004 and 2013—were due to "adverse events related to dietary supplements."

Laxatives in Your St. John's Wort?

A 2015 Canadian study tested popular herbal supplements and found that many of the bottles contained pills that were diluted or contained none of the product listed on the label. Others consisted entirely of fillers such as soybeans, wheat, and rice—ingredients that were not necessarily on the label. These were the only "plants" in the pill. One bottle of St. John's wort, the *New York Times* reported, "contained only Alexandrian senna, an Egyptian yellow shrub that is a powerful laxative." Other supplements contained walnuts, potentially deadly for people with nut allergies. This study suggests that the problem may be widespread. It is especially troubling for those with a severe food allergy or requiring a strict gluten-free diet.

This study and others prompted the New York State attorney general in 2015 to issue a cease-and-desist order to several large chains selling supplements, requiring them to withdraw the products. He was joined by other state agencies. The aim of the initiative is to require manufacturers to address their own product issues so that supplements are not pulled from store shelves *after* they have done harm.

If you are currently gluten-free and suddenly have a return of symptoms, you may need to look at the supplements you take instead of what you had for dinner the night before. Unfortunately, inspecting the label may not help—the "FACTS" section of a supplement label may show the product contains very little or none of this important "ingredient."

Another study published in the *Journal of the American Medical Association* found that half of the FDA Class I recalls between 2008 and 2012—where there is a "reasonable probability that [their use] will cause serious adverse health consequences or death"—were supplements. And about two-thirds of the recalled dietary supplements that were analyzed still contained banned drugs at least six months after being recalled. These banned and/or prescription-only drugs found in supplements included:

- **Sibutramine**—a weight-loss drug that was withdrawn from the U.S. market in October 2010 since it is known to substantially increase blood pressure and/or pulse rate and may present a significant risk of heart attack and stroke in some people.
- **Sildenafil**—used for erectile dysfunction, it can cause hearing loss and low blood pressure and reacts with a number of other prescription drugs.
- **Fluoxetine**—trade name Prozac, this drug is sold only by prescription.
- **Phenolphthalein**—formerly the main component in laxatives, such as Ex-Lax, banned by the FDA in 1999 for sale in the U.S. due to the risk of causing cancer with long-term use.
- **Aromatase inhibitor**—used by prescription only in breast cancer treatments to lower estrogen levels.
- **Various anabolic steroids.**

A September 2015 recall by the FDA is particularly sobering. Two weight loss supplements were found to contain both sibutramine and phenolphthalein—neither of which were listed on the label. They were marketed under the names Pink Bikini and Shorts on the Beach and sold online. The FDA also noted that "these products may also interact in life-threatening ways with other medications a consumer may be taking."

Most of the FDA-recalled supplements were for bodybuilding, weight loss, and sexual enhancement. If you use these products, you may be getting an enhancement in the form of side effects you did not bargain for. Supplement labels may hide more than that pink bikini can.

When Your Doctor Advises Vitamin or Mineral Supplements

Vitamin deficiencies are often found in people with newly diagnosed celiac disease and require supplementation until the gut has healed and can absorb nutrients properly, and the deficiency is resolved. Anyone on a restricted diet or with another GI condition that involves malabsorption is also a candidate for supplementation.

We recommend choosing a gluten-free vitamin that has only the regulated amounts of vitamins. Try to avoid multivitamins that have megadoses of anything.

People who eat processed food are most likely getting their vitamins synthetically to begin with. Milk, fortified with vitamin D, is the primary source of D for most people who avoid the sun. Ironically, cereals, breads, flours, and canned foods all are fortified to replace the vitamins and minerals removed by processing. But manufacturers have just begun to fortify gluten-free foods, and this can pose problems for someone who has grown accustomed to obtaining their vitamins synthetically from processed food and is now on a gluten-free diet.

The pendulum can easily swing in the other direction. Many people still take megadoses of vitamins, assuming that if some is good, more must be better. We see more people with vitamin B6 toxicity than deficiency, due to excess supplementation.

Vitamin B6 (pyridoxine) is involved in many metabolic functions throughout the body. It is needed for brain development and function and involved in the process of making serotonin and norepinephrine, chemical transmitters in the brain. Although vitamin B6 is often promoted for "nervous system health," its toxicity is usually focused on the nervous system. A vitamin B6 deficiency is rare in the general population since it is found in many foods.

Test First

It is not surprising that many people, anxious about the amount of different vitamins they are getting in their diet, rely so heavily on vitamin and mineral supplements. What *is* surprising is that they read the pros and ignore the cons—the toxicities, interactions with other vitamins and drugs, contamination, and mislabeling.

A vitamin or mineral deficiency can be ascertained by blood tests and addressed by some simple dietary changes.

A Word on Fatigue and L-Carnitine

L-carnitine is an amino acid that is produced by the body and a natural component of the diet. It helps the body produce energy and is used in Europe to treat fatigue and as a replacement supplement for people on a very strict vegetarian/vegan diet.

It is found in high levels in red meat and in lower levels in dairy products as well as pork, seafood, and chicken. High levels of carnitine are found in those who consume excess amounts of red meat. A natural compound, it is available by prescription as well as over the counter.

L-carnitine excess can cause a number of side effects including diarrhea, nausea, and cramps. It can interact with prescription drugs and is associated with increased risk of cardiovascular disease. You should take supplements only under a doctor's instruction. (See chapter 17, "Celiac Disease.")

Widely Used Supplements That Cause Drug Interactions

We don't want to focus on the trees (or their leaves) at the expense of the forest.

—DOUGLAS R. HOFSTADTER, PROFESSOR OF COGNITIVE SCIENCE

Recently several large studies have examined the contents of various supplements. Many were tested and found to contain allergens, little or none of the herb or vitamin on the label, or a banned substance. Others are potentially dangerous in their interaction with common medications. A few are worth mentioning.

St. John's Wort

St. John's wort is one of the 10 best-selling supplements in the U.S. It is marketed as a mood elevator and is arguably the most popular supplement to treat depression. But St. John's wort can speed the breakdown of various prescription medicines by eliminating them from the body before they can take full effect. This includes anticoagulants (blood thinners), oral contraceptives, antidepressants, cancer drugs, and immunosuppressants (causing transplant rejection).

Vitamin K

Vitamin K helps in blood coagulation but in excess can block the effect of medications like warfarin (blood thinners) used to prevent blood clots. Because it is now added to many calcium supplements and found in multivitamins, it can quietly reach high levels in the body and trigger problems before someone is aware of any issue.

Vitamin C

Vitamin C will facilitate iron absorption. People with a tendency to absorb excess iron should be careful with this supplement.

Zinc

Taken by many to "shorten a cold," zinc has numerous GI side effects and interacts with antibiotics and antihypertensive medications.

Ginseng

Used in Chinese medicine for heart issues, this is another popular herb that can interfere with anticoagulant drugs like warfarin and can interact with some antidepressant medications. It has been implicated in neonatal death when taken by the mother.

The list is long. Licorice, black cohosh, echinacea, ginkgo, and many of the most popular herbs are the subject of questionable claims, drug interactions, and lack of quality control.

You should limit vitamin intake to the vitamins you are deficient in— validated through testing and as directed by your doctor.

Supplements for Those Age 50 and Up

While taking supplements can be harmful at any age, older adults are more likely to encounter problems. Older adults also usually take more and a wider variety of prescription drugs than younger people, and this increases the risk of a dangerous interaction with supplements. In addition, many patients do not tell their doctors about the nonprescription pills they ingest, and many doctors do not ask about them—leading to potentially serious consequences.

Supplements, like many prescription drugs, are metabolized and eliminated through the kidney and liver. Since older people have higher rates of kidney and/or liver disease, it may be harder for their body to process compounds found in supplements. The interactions with the cardiovascular system can be particularly problematic. Taking blood thinners or cardiovascular drugs with St. John's wort, vitamin K, zinc, or ginseng may cause serious problems.

Probiotic Intoxication

We think, each of us, that we're much more rational than we are.
And we think that we make our decisions because we have good
reasons to make them. Even when it's the other way around. We
believe in the reasons, because we've already made the decision.
—DANIEL KAHNEMAN, PSYCHOLOGIST AND
BEHAVIORAL ECONOMIST, NOBEL LAUREATE

Probiotic is the term currently used to name the live bacteria/microorganisms taken by people to supposedly correct and/or maintain the natural balance of their gut and microbiome. This raises the question of what is a "natural" and "healthy" balance of microbiota—proportions that science has not yet been able to determine.

The balance of different bacteria varies from person to person, as well as culture to culture, depending on eating habits, genes, and environment. And while we know that a diverse microbiome is desirable, not everyone needs "rebalancing" to stay healthy.

A recent study of a tribe of hunter-gatherers in Africa, the Hadza people of Tanzania, showed that they lacked *Bifidobacterium*, a bacterium that is found in probiotic foods and considered healthy. They also had other bacteria that are considered a sign of disease in Western populations.

The study underscores the need to redefine what is healthy and unhealthy in our microbiota and how different bacteria interact with each other. And more important, that a far more personalized approach to probiotics is needed if they are to be effectively utilized to treat human health.

Manipulating the gut microbiota may prove to be an effective way to control the development of diseases and influence treatment. While the benefits of probiotics are being actively studied, it is still scientifically unclear whether they work for specific diseases. You are consuming live bacteria with the assumption that it is a "good" versus "bad" bacteria. For those taking probiotics during antibiotic therapy, how do you know that the antibiotic is not killing the probiotic you are taking or interfering with its action? Probiotics are regulated as a food, not a drug. Which means that they are largely unregulated. They need to be reported to your doctor along with any pharmaceuticals that you are taking.

More important, the safety of their use by young children, older adults, and anyone with a compromised or weak immune system is unclear and potentially dangerous.

While many people have had symptomatic relief through the use of probiotics, the health claims related to these products are often questionable and derived from animal studies that may not translate to humans, as well as studies of different types of bacteria (e.g., lactobacilli and bifidobacteria) that have huge differences within each species. For example, there are 170 species of *Lactobacillus*, one of the most widely advertised and available probiotic bacterium. All are part of the normal gastrointestinal and vaginal flora and are used in a variety of commercial products. Yet only some strains have been tested; others lack any real data.

While probiotics are being tested in the treatment of many different medical conditions (allergies, obesity, liver disease, IBS, diarrhea caused by antibiotics, and stomach ulcers, to name a few), it is still too early to know if they are truly effective or safe for these conditions, though studies in irritable bowel syndrome look promising.

The Upside—Some Studies Are Very Promising

Some probiotics digest or alter gluten. One commercially available probiotic that contains eight different bacteria can reduce the toxicity of gluten when used in a fermentation process. A study of sourdough baked wheat products fermented by specific bacteria and funguses was shown to be safe for people with celiac disease.

Probiotics cannot at this point be recommended for the pharmaceutical treatment of celiac disease as they have not as yet been proven safe and effective, but they are an exciting area of research.

Clostridium Difficile and Fecal Transplants

Fecal transplants and certain probiotics have been proven to be effective in combating *Clostridium difficile* (also called *C. difficile* and *C. diff*)—a potentially deadly infection—especially its recurrence. This bacterial infection, formerly found mainly in older populations, causes diarrhea and inflammation of the colon and is increasing in younger people.

Fecal microbiota transplant is a procedure where fecal matter (stool) is collected from a healthy donor and transplanted into the affected patient, usually during a colonoscopy. The theory is to replace "good" bacteria that has been killed or suppressed by *C. difficile* overrunning the colon. The transplant is essentially repopulating a disturbed microbiota and—while still classified as experimental—appears extremely effective for this life-threatening condition. There are now capsules of stool extract available, and hopefully the research on the use of specific bacteria will make this therapy more palatable.

Using one kind of "natural" bacteria to combat another is well studied in this condition, and the offending pathogen is well known. This practice cannot be automatically translated to the treatment of other conditions. Researchers do not yet know which strains to select for specific physical and clinical conditions, the effect of different doses, or the effect on mechanisms or function.

Patients have reported weight gain and mood changes after receiving stool from overweight and/or "unhappy" donors. While this feedback may be anecdotal, there is some research linking changes in the microbiome and weight gain. (See chapter 9, "The Microbiome.")

The Downside—Quality Control

A 2015 study at the Center tested 22 probiotic products purchased commercially and examined them for gluten. About 30 percent of them had some form of gluten that was not listed on the label. As a result, we feel that supplement labels claiming a product is gluten-free cannot currently be trusted.

This in some ways reconfirms a previous study we did showing that patients with celiac disease who regularly took supplements had more symptoms than those who did not take supplements. Interestingly, they also reported a higher quality of life. This may attest to the placebo effect of supplements—they make people better because we expect them to. The "action" would appear to be more brain than gut.

It is unclear whether the levels of gluten found in the probiotics tested posed a risk to people with celiac disease, but the results reflect the underlying problem of supplement oversight, regulation, labeling, and testing.

Are the Products Viable?

Over-the-counter pills may not be a viable source of live bacteria. The probiotics in food (yogurts and acidified milks in cold storage) are usually produced with stricter control and contain viable amounts if stored properly and consumed before the expiration date.

Like other supplements, probiotics are produced and labeled with little oversight from the FDA or other agencies that guard consumer health interests. **The consumer is currently not buying the carefully regulated probiotic mixtures used in research studies.**

Reading Labels—"Doctor Recommended"?

"You see what you expect to see, Severus."
—ALBUS DUMBLEDORE IN J. K. ROWLING'S *HARRY POTTER AND THE DEATHLY HALLOWS*

Unethical marketing claims abound in supplement advertisements. Word-of-mouth endorsements coupled with aggressive advertising on every form of traditional and social media have fueled the supplement boom. Great examples are the products marketed as digesting gluten—a claim that is blatantly false. The pharmaceutical industry is currently developing and testing enzymes that *will* digest the toxic fragments of gluten that cause celiac disease, but none of the currently available products do this. (See chapter 30, "Nondietary Therapies.")

The brain-gut connection is quite clear: We want to believe the claims, and some people actually feel better on supplements. This may be a placebo effect, but that has not been well studied. Unfortunately, supplements make many people sick from trying to correct conditions they never had.

Until we understand the composition, diversity, function, metabolic capacity, and plasticity of the microbial communities within us, attempting to manipulate them will continue to be somewhat hit-or-miss.

A Word of Advice

Real estate agents always advise: location, location, location. The microbes that inhabit the mouth are different from those found in the stomach, the small intestine, and the large intestine. Therefore, if microbes are to be studied in terms of their communication with the brain and body, researchers must first determine which bacteria and which gut area to target in any given therapy.

By inserting one type of bacteria to knock out another, what else is being destroyed or affected? The human gastrointestinal tract is a bacterial ecosystem with a genetic makeup almost 100 times the size of the human genome. We are therefore an amalgam of both our human genes and microbial "selves." And the interaction of the two is largely unexplored territory. Probiotics are an exciting area of research but should be ingested with great caution.

> *There are 3 billion base pairs of nucleotides in the human genome engaged in a vast and complex dance that makes us who we are. We need to be awfully careful when we start to change the choreography, especially given our current lack of precision. When you try to move one dancer with a bulldozer, you're pretty darn certain to scoop up more than one Rockette.*
> —DR. SHARON MOALEM, *SURVIVAL OF THE SICKEST*

Summary

Supplements are overused and understudied regarding their effectiveness and safety. It is an industry that advertises heavily but lacks thorough regulatory oversight and quality control. Heavy metals, banned animal, pharmaceutical, and plant products, steroids, untested ingredients, and prescription medications are found in various supplements.

While prescription drugs must be proven safe and effective before they are marketed, probiotics and other dietary supplements do not need to pass that test. Every year contents are withdrawn because of toxicity—after the fact. One case report of a death in a child due to contamination with a fungus is enough to dampen enthusiasm.

As a 2014 news item from Columbia University noted: "This year marks the 20th anniversary of the passage of one of the most skillful pieces of legislation ever to undermine the health of Americans: the Dietary Supplement Health and Educational Act of 1994. The result was to remove from regulation by the Food and Drug Administration any substances labeled as a dietary supplement." It is time to take a hard look at the various vitamin, mineral, and probiotics bottles in your "medicine" cabinet and on your kitchen counter. Be well advised that you may be flushing money—quite literally—down the toilet and, more important, jeopardizing your health. Too many people are taking supplements and probiotics while removing the foods that naturally contain these vitamins and minerals from their diets.

While some dietary and medical supplementation is useful, much of it simply reflects media trends that we can enhance and increase our health with a fix-it pill. It is as enticing as it is unrealistic.

Natural does not mean safe.

6

A Word on Testing—What Do Antibodies Tell Us?

Test first, then you treat right.
—NORTH AMERICAN SOCIETY FOR THE
STUDY OF CELIAC DISEASE

Many people complain that they are "simply lab results" to their doctors. But these tests are often the most effective way of finding—as well as ruling out—serious conditions and avoiding complications. Rushing to self-diagnose gastrointestinal distress can mask a serious condition or prolong symptoms that can be cured if recognized and treated medically. Lab tests cannot resolve every issue, and they can lead to false conclusions, but they can quickly pinpoint and/or eliminate the causes of many GI complaints.

Since the GI tract is difficult to see without invasive procedures, various blood and breath tests can explain why some people do not respond to a gluten-free diet, why a drug may not cure a symptom—or cause others—and help to identify actual vitamin and mineral deficiencies. They enabled us to diagnose Carol's drug-induced hepatitis before it caused serious complications and permanent liver damage. (See chapter 5, "Supplements and Probiotics.")

Diagnostic tests for specific conditions are described in the following chapters, but it is important for anyone suffering from GI symptoms that they feel are caused by or related to gluten to understand the basic tests used to facilitate a diagnosis. What you see and feel may be the tip of a hidden iceberg, and a gluten-free diet may not help you avoid the impact of a collision.

Rule Out Celiac Disease

If you are suffering from symptoms that include:

- chronic diarrhea or constipation
- gas/bloating
- anemia
- vomiting
- canker sores
- weight loss
- failure to thrive (in children)
- vitamin deficiencies
- lactose intolerance
- behavioral issues
- brain fog
- neuropathies

and/or celiac disease has been diagnosed in a family member, you should be tested for celiac disease *before* starting a gluten-free diet. Once you are on the diet, testing becomes more difficult to interpret, can be inaccurate, and may require a gluten challenge that brings a return of unwanted symptoms.

The blood and endoscopic tests for celiac disease are detailed in chapter 17. These are the definitive tests to determine if someone is mounting an autoimmune reaction to gluten that is destroying the lining of their small intestine and interfering with digestion.

Get Basic Standard of Care Tests

If you have continuing GI symptoms, it is important to know if your gut/ body is inflamed, if you are anemic, and to measure specific vitamins and minerals to assess for the presence and severity of malabsorption. These tests also help your doctor to determine what part(s) of the intestine are involved and the degree of damage.

Tests include:

- **Erythrocyte sedimentation rate and C-reactive protein**— reveals the degree of inflammation in the body; they are not specific for any particular condition or organ.
- **Ferritin**—a parameter of iron stores, inflammation, or deficiency due to malabsorption or chronic blood loss. High values reflect excessive iron stores, as in hemochromatosis, a genetic disorder of excessive iron absorption that is associated with celiac disease.
- **Folic acid**—a parameter of disease of the upper small intestine, where it is absorbed. A deficiency or low levels are common in celiac disease and rare in Crohn's disease, which is predominantly in the ileum or lower small intestine.
- **B12**—a parameter of lower small intestinal disease or stomach issues such as bacterial overgrowth or chronic gastritis.
- **Vitamin D**—necessary for calcium absorption (in turn, necessary for bone formation and muscle contraction). Vitamin D is formed in the skin from sun exposure that can be impeded by sunblock and lack of outdoor activity. Dietary deficiency is also common.
- **Parathyroid hormone**—the parathyroid monitors and manages calcium metabolism. With calcium deficiency, the hormone increases to retain calcium and maintain blood levels to ensure cardiac, blood, and muscle function.

- **Stool testing**—important in GI issues to look for blood and, with diarrhea, to look for infections.

If there are neurological issues, vitamins E, B1, B2, and B6 as well as copper levels should be measured. If there are skin rashes or taste issues, zinc should be measured.

Use Breath Tests to Further Narrow the Diagnosis

Breath tests are used to diagnose a number of conditions that produce GI symptoms, including fructose and lactose intolerance, bacterial overgrowth, and intestinal transit time. It is important to exclude these conditions in patients with irritable bowel syndrome (IBS) and celiac disease with persistent symptoms.

The sugars and carbohydrates we eat are normally digested and absorbed in the small intestine. But when they are mal-absorbed, they get into the colon, where they are fermented by the bacteria that live there. The bacteria dine happily on them, producing gas, water, and the painful symptoms known to those suffering from IBS. This also produces the hydrogen and/or methane gas that are a normal by-product of carbohydrate digestion. These gases are absorbed into the bloodstream and eliminated through the lungs in the breath.

Patients drink different sugars (sucrose, glucose, lactulose, fructose), and their breath is measured every half hour with special analyzers in order to measure the "peaks" of hydrogen and to determine if and how rapidly you are absorbing or mal-absorbing sugars. If lactose and fructose are digested and absorbed in the small intestine, you normally will not produce excess hydrogen.

Therefore, an increase in hydrogen indicates specific intestinal problems. With rapid transit, hydrogen is produced soon after the sugar is ingested; with bacterial overgrowth, hydrogen levels peak twice—once when digested by bacteria not normally found in the small intestine and later by the bacteria in the colon.

Breath tests are a simple and safe method of measuring alterations in digestion that create symptoms, but they have limitations. Some people have colon bacteria that produce methane gas instead of hydrogen, while others produce both. Patterns of release vary from patient to patient—some people have slower but normal transit time. Other conditions may produce malabsorption of carbohydrates, such as pancreatic insufficiency and celiac disease.

Breath tests can be particularly helpful for people with IBS told to go on the FODMAP diet. They can help to eliminate specific problem carbohydrates prior to starting a very restrictive diet. If you can isolate the main carbohydrate problem you can eliminate many weeks of trial and error. The tests should be part of a gastroenterologist's armamentarium but are often not widely available or utilized.

Test for Vitamin and Mineral Deficiencies

My husband does not eat anything that is orange, green, or yellow—otherwise known as vegetables. He'll eat tomatoes because I told him they were fruit.

(TESS, 29)

Many people take vitamin and mineral supplements because they make them feel healthier. Others use them to supplement a restrictive diet. Several websites and TV personalities suggest easy ways to determine if you are deficient in specific vitamins. One "analysis" includes standing on your right foot for three seconds without losing your balance (to diagnose a B12 deficiency), or pressing your thumb into your breastbone to see if this causes discomfort (to diagnose a vitamin D deficiency). This "testing" ranges from useless to preposterous. It is more likely to uncover a balance disorder and/or leave a black-and-blue mark from pressing too hard.

If you feel that your diet does not contain sufficient amounts of everything your body needs, have your doctor run blood tests for essential vitamins and minerals.

While there are many people in the world suffering from malnutrition and serious vitamin deficiencies, they are rarely the people buying supplements in health food stores. People with malabsorption conditions—celiac disease, inflammatory bowel disease, protein allergies, intestinal damage, etc.—need to be monitored and, if necessary, supplemented, but a balanced diet of fresh ingredients is usually adequate to supply what the body requires.

For better or worse, our diets contain a surplus of fortified foods that usually make up for the nutrients removed during the processing that extends shelf life. An overuse of many vitamins can lead to toxicity, drug interactions, and other serious problems.

What Do Antibodies to Gluten Really Mean?

> When the right thing can only be measured poorly, it tends
> to cause the wrong thing to be measured well. And it is often
> much worse to have a good measurement of the wrong thing,
> especially when it is so often the case that the wrong thing
> will, in fact, be used as an indicator of [what is] right.
>
> —JOHN TUKEY, PROMINENT STATISTICIAN

In the following chapters—notably those in Part V, which examine several psychiatric and neurological conditions—we refer to "antigliadin antibodies" that are found in the bloodstream of people with these disorders. While not part of current standard-of-care testing, they are the focus of many research studies on gut-brain interactions, and therefore a quick primer on immunoglobulins is in order.

What Do Antibodies Do?

Antibodies (also known as immunoglobulins) are a critical component of the immune system. They can do many things:

- Recognize and bind to a target and inactivate or destroy it
- Attract other cells when they do bind
- Set in motion a number of immune functions
- Initiate a cascade of other chemicals
- Cross-link other molecules

Antibodies are designed to recognize and neutralize toxins in the body by inactivating bacteria and viral products. They may also inappropriately recognize and react with specific "self" proteins. So, developed by nature to fight infection, they then fight us. The by-product is autoimmunity.

Antibodies to gluten (antigliadin antibodies or AGA) are targeting gliadin, the protein portion of gluten. They are markers that indicate an abnormal immune system response to gluten in people with celiac disease but are not specific for the disease. They have, however, been seen in the blood of some patients with autism spectrum disorder (ASD), attention deficit hyperactivity disorder (ADHD), schizophrenia, and cerebral palsy. These are *not* celiac antibodies, and the significance of this immune response has not yet been explained.

Immunoglobulin Primer

Antibodies/immunoglobulins (Ig) are classified by their specific features, structure, targets, and locations. Important to our discussion are:

IgA—antibodies that are found throughout the GI tract and other body surfaces that are exposed to the environment and foreign substances. They deal with surface and mucosal immunity and are seen in celiac disease.

IgE—antibodies that circulate in the bloodstream and trigger the immediate immune response in an allergic reaction. They are present in much smaller quantities than the other major classes. Allergies are IgE mediated: When IgE antibodies bind to pollen, venom, dander, or food antigens they cause the release of histamines that trigger symptoms such as swollen airways and other reactions found in food allergies.

IgG—the most common in the body, they fight bacterial and viral infections. They are the only antibodies that can cross the placenta. They are also seen in food sensitivities.

Both IgA and IgG antibodies recognize and react to gluten. IgG antigliadin antibodies are found in some people with autism spectrum disorder, ADHD, schizophrenia, and cerebral palsy. IgG antigliadin antibodies are also found in the bloodstream of healthy people.

If some patients with psychiatric and neurological conditions have antigliadin antibodies, they may be the best candidates to benefit from a gluten-free diet. However, we do not know if the antibodies develop due to an intestinal issue or are the result of the neuropsychiatric condition influencing intestinal function. Also, the gut-brain axis may be bidirectional.

The presence of antigliadin antibodies must be shown to have a direct effect on function to be considered significant. At this point, the direct effect on neural function of antigliadin antibodies is still being debated. If it is possible to eliminate these antibodies through a strict gluten-free diet, it may have important therapeutic implications, though this has not been demonstrated. It is still unclear if these antigliadin antibodies are cause, effect, or simply innocent bystanders.

"Nonsense on Stilts" Testing

Tennis superstar Novak Djokovic was supposedly diagnosed by a doctor who was a family friend by putting a slice of bread on his stomach and holding up his arm as the doctor pushed against it.* While Djokovic felt it was "madness," he noticed a difference in his ability to resist the pressure. This form of kinesiology is not reliable or accepted testing. As writer Alex Gazzola noted, "I cannot help but wonder how a top athlete can come to be convinced of this stuff. 'What matters is that you are open-minded' is Djokovic's take. Yes—but not so open-minded that your brains fall out." A gluten-free diet has apparently changed Djokovic's game and life, but his diagnostic journey is not a medical testing game changer.

Summary

Issues need to be isolated if they are to be properly diagnosed and a patient is to find treatment and relief. Because the gastrointestinal symptoms of different disorders mimic one another, it is intuitively easy to point a finger at the wrong food or event as a trigger. Diarrhea and pain can be caused by a bacterial infection, a virus, food poisoning, carbohydrate intolerance, lactose intolerance, celiac disease, or acute pancreatitis, as well as a long list of other multisystem disorders.

Test first, test right, and treat right.

---

* Reported in an article in the *Wall Street Journal*.

PART II

What Is Going On in the Gut

(The Science Basics)

Nature uses only the longest threads to weave her patterns, so that each small piece of her fabric reveals the organization of the entire tapestry.
—RICHARD FEYNMAN, PHYSICIST

There is a game called "telephone" in which one person starts a message that is whispered from one participant to another until the last person in the game announces the final message and the person who started the game states the original. Usually, the message announced by the final person is totally different and only bizarrely connected to the original. It is a game that shows how small misconceptions can make a huge difference, how errors accumulate.

What goes on in your gut is a bit like the game telephone. Foods, drugs, and supplements interact with many participants in the digestive process, and a crossed signal, misinterpreted message, or inflamed surface changes the effect of that food or drug into a cascade of unexpected problems for the body. The original intent is often lost in the translation.

The gut is a complex and intricate system composed of different organs, glands, enzymes, secretions, cells, and nerves as well as trillions of bacteria, viruses, fungi, and yeast that compose the microbiome. It also has its very own "second brain." There are many places for communications to go awry when every element is getting and sending whispered messages.

The Normal Gut and Digestion

The human body is a machine which winds its own springs.
—JULIEN OFFROY DE LA METTRIE,
18TH-CENTURY PHYSICIAN AND PHILOSOPHER

I don't digest things with my mind.
—MARILYN MONROE

In many ways, the digestive system is an extension of the environment—a long tube, open at both ends, that is designed to supply the body with all the nutrients and fluids it needs to function. And everything we consume—food, liquids, drugs, supplements, Play-Doh—ultimately affects the entire body as it travels through the tract.

Digestion is an amazingly effective and efficient process. The concept is simple, the design and execution quite remarkable and, as scientists are discovering, intriguingly complex. There is a constant interaction of organs, muscles, nerves, hormones, enzymes, microbes, and blood vessels, every one doing tasks that monitor, regulate, and control the job of nourishing the body. As you will see, our gut goes well beyond simply processing the food we eat. It engages in a constant conversation with other parts of the body. And the volume is often deafening.

Problems in the digestive tract are one of the most common reasons people seek medical help—or self-medicate with restrictive diets, over-the-counter remedies, supplements, and/or pre- and probiotics. The list is long, and the discomfort and inconvenience of gastrointestinal distress a source of pain as well as embarrassment.

To understand what goes wrong, and the real basis of GI problems, it is important to understand first how digestion actually occurs. It is an essential foundation for comprehending how what we ingest affects both body and brain, and why going gluten-free or lactose-free or carbohydrate-free works for some and not for others. And why we were not meant to simply eliminate one category of nutrients without ample cause.

> I spend a great deal of time on the toilet. In fact, I do some of my best work in the bathroom.
>
> (ED, 44, CROHN'S DISEASE)

The Gastrointestinal Tract

Since nothing we eat can be used by the body in its ingested form, digestion is a combination of mechanical and chemical processes that tear food apart, grind it down, shake it vigorously, and create a soupy mix that is propelled through the entire length of the digestive tract (the gut), where it is ultimately absorbed and anything unusable is eliminated.

Food enters the mouth, where it is chewed into smaller pieces and enzymes begin digestion. It then travels through the pharynx, esophagus, stomach, small intestine (the duodenum, jejunum, and ileum), and large intestine (colon), and nondigestible products exit from the anus. Throughout the GI tract are organs and glands—salivary glands, pancreas, liver, and gallbladder—that secrete the enzymes and fluids needed to break down and digest food.

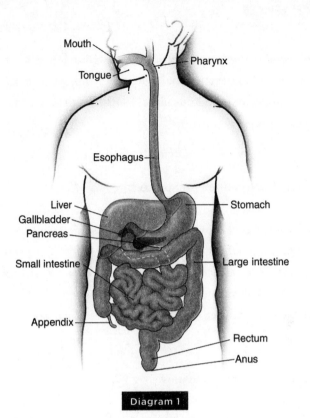

Diagram 1

THE DIGESTIVE TRACT

The digestive system is intimately joined to:

- the circulatory system, which supplies nutrients to the organs and other tissues throughout the body
- the enteric (intrinsic) and autonomic (automatic) nervous systems, which control enzyme release and contractions of the gut, and report back to the brain
- the muscles of the digestive system, which provide coordinated motility (movement) to help digest and move/squeeze food through the long tract
- the hormones that regulate movement as well as the secretions that stimulate and/or inhibit the activities of digestion

While there is enormous capacity and redundancy built into the digestive system, if one section malfunctions, it almost necessarily affects another, and there are numerous places for things to go wrong.

Digestion

Digestion is actually a three-part process:

1. **Digestion**—the breakdown of food products into smaller components that can be absorbed.
2. **Absorption**—the passage of food products that have been broken down into the intestinal wall.
3. **Transport**—the transfer of food from the intestinal wall to the rest of the body.

It consists of two basic activities:

- the **mechanical** chewing and mixing of food in the mouth and stomach and propulsion by the intestinal muscle, called *peristalsis*. This muscular component is a crucial aspect of digestion since contractions of the smooth muscle both propel and mix the chyme (the liquid product of the broken-down food) as it travels down the digestive tract. Without peristalsis, there would be no digestion. When we discuss a lack of motility in various GI conditions, it means that peristalsis is affected.
- the **chemical** breakdown of food by secretions and enzymes throughout the digestive tract. This starts with saliva in the mouth and is completed by microbes in the colon.

Digestion actually begins before the food even enters your mouth. When you see, think about, or smell food, the *vagus nerve* transmits a chemical message from your brain to release saliva in the mouth, increase stomach movement, and release gastric acid in the stomach. You begin to salivate, and the stomach "rumbles" at the very anticipation of food.

The Mouth

Digestion starts in the mouth as chewing tears, grinds, and crushes the food into smaller pieces. Saliva is secreted by glands under and around the tongue to lubricate and start to dissolve the food. Saliva contains enzymes that begin the digestion of fats and carbohydrates and acts as a glue to hold the food together as it travels toward the stomach.

The nervous system lends a hand to this process by inhibiting as well as stimulating the release of saliva. This is why we often get a "dry mouth" when fearful, and salivate at the thought or smell of food when hungry.

We swallow the ball or *bolus* of chewed food and saliva that is transported down our esophagus. While the skeletal muscles at work in the mouth and throat are voluntary—we consciously move our jaws and swallow—smooth muscles that function involuntarily then take over in the esophagus. This is where peristalsis begins and moves the food into the stomach, where the action really begins.

The Stomach

The stomach is a big muscular bag that holds the chewed food, mixes it with gastric juices, and starts many of the chemical processes of digestion. The muscle movements of the stomach act like a Cuisinart—chopping, blending, and mixing the ball of food into a soupy puree called *chyme.*

The main chemical ingredient in the stomach is hydrochloric (gastric) acid, a highly corrosive substance that both breaks down the food and converts the stomach into a disinfecting tank, killing bacteria and toxins in the food we have eaten. Gastric acid is an essential line of defense in the body's monitoring of dangerous substances entering it from the outside. The stomach also releases *pepsin,* an enzyme that digests protein.

The walls of the stomach are composed of several layers of tissue—a structure found throughout the rest of the GI tract—that contain numerous mucous glands able to secrete mucus into the tract to lubricate the lining and protect it from friction and the acid bath of the chyme. The breakdown of this mucus coating is one of the causes of ulcers.

The communication system in the stomach also sends hormonal messages to the other digestive organs that food has arrived. This stimulates the secretion of pancreatic juices and bile from the liver that will further break down the chyme once it moves into the small intestine.

One-Way Street

Food is only meant to travel *down* the GI tract—a street sign that is often ignored. The sphincters (ring-like muscles) connecting the esophagus to the stomach and the stomach to the small intestine are one-way valves. Occasionally, chyme refluxes or backs up into the esophageal area—a condition known as GERD, gastroesophageal reflux disease. The corrosive effect of gastric acid is well known to people who experience its effect on their less-well-protected esophagus. (See chapter 8, "The Gut in Disease.")

When the chyme is sufficiently liquefied, muscle/peristaltic contractions gradually push it into the upper part of the small intestine, the duodenum. The stomach empties in a slow and controlled way so as not to overwhelm all the mechanisms of digestion in the small intestine. Everything is released according to particle size.

As the small intestine fills with chyme, it signals the stomach to decrease its activity and slow down the emptying process. This is one reason a large or fatty meal stays with you. It lingers in the stomach until the small intestine is ready to process it.

The arrival of chyme in the small intestine triggers the release of a cascade of secretions. The small intestine, pancreas, liver, and gallbladder all deliver digestive enzymes and fluids that break down the food into components small enough to be absorbed. Alkaline mucus with a high concentration of bicarbonate is secreted to neutralize the gastric acid in the chyme.

All of these actions are regulated by both the nervous system and gastrointestinal hormones and called into action only when needed by the digestive system.

Most of these activities occur without any conscious awareness or control. In this sense, it is truly a "second brain" in your gut.

The Pancreas

A carrot-shaped gland that has a dual function in digestion and metabolism, the pancreas is both an endocrine gland—producing insulin, which enables the digestion and absorption of carbohydrates—and an exocrine gland—producing enzymes such as trypsin, which breaks down proteins; *amylase*, which breaks down starches; and *lipase*, which breaks down fats. When the pancreas becomes inflamed or diseased (e.g., pancreatitis), these enzymes are not secreted, and as a result carbohydrate, protein, and fat digestion is impaired.

The Liver

The liver is the energy-processing center of the body. It is the first stop for nutrients absorbed from the intestine. Its many functions include metabolizing, storing, and transporting nutrients to the body, producing chemicals necessary for digestion, and breaking down drugs and alcohol.

The liver stores glucose, iron, and vitamins A, B12, and D, sending out the nutrients and substances digested from the food to the cells of the body as they are needed. It also secretes bile, a fluid that increases the solubility of fats, enabling them to pass through the intestinal wall into the bloodstream. Bile is made in the liver and stored in the gallbladder until needed, and delivered to the small intestine when fatty foods arrive and stimulate its release through contraction of the gallbladder.

The Small Intestine

The small intestine, which is actually the longest part of the GI tract, is designed to complete digestion and much of the absorption of nutrients. It is approximately 22 feet long in adults and consists of three parts:

- the duodenum (the first segment)
- jejunum (the second segment)
- ileum (the third segment, or distal small intestine)

All three segments have similar anatomy, but each has a specialized job, digesting and absorbing specific nutrients.

Slow waves of peristalsis push chyme from the stomach through the duodenum toward the jejunum. It actually takes several hours for an entire meal to travel the entire length of the small intestine to enable absorption to occur through the lining or mucosal wall of the intestine.

This lining has a unique structure that possesses a much larger surface area than the midsection of the body in which it is contained. (See Diagram 2.) This lining, the *mucosa*, consists of folds that increase its surface area. The folds are in turn covered with tiny fingerlike projections, or *villi*, that contain the cells that absorb nutrients and again expand the surface area. (See Diagram 3.)

The surface of each villus has a "brush" border consisting of *microvilli* or tiny hairs that increase the absorptive surface of the small intestine yet again. The brush border also secretes enzymes that are necessary for the digestion of specific food components.

If you were to flatten out the intestinal mucosa—all the villi, microvilli, and crypts that lie between the villi—the "small" intestine actually has a surface area about the size of a football field that is totally dedicated to absorbing food! This enormous capacity ensures that the intestine can sustain a fair amount of assault and/or damage and still feed the body.

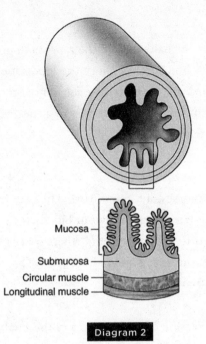

Mucosa
Submucosa
Circular muscle
Longitudinal muscle

Diagram 2

A CROSS SECTION OF THE INTESTINAL WALL

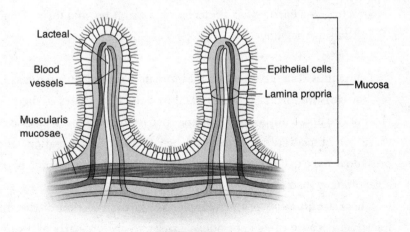

Lacteal

Blood
vessels

Muscularis
mucosae

Epithelial cells

Lamina propria

Mucosa

Diagram 3

Inflammatory cells normally inhabit the mucosa to protect the small intestine against toxins and bacteria. Since the food supply entering the GI tract is not sterile and may contain toxic substances, these white blood cells are another line of defense. This results in a state of constant, controlled inflammation in the mucosa.

The Villi

The villi are the workhorses of the intestine. They are the final intestinal link between your dinner plate and your bloodstream. This is where celiac disease does its primary damage and where other gluten and food-related disorders affect the body's ability to properly absorb nutrients.

The villi play a crucial role by:

- dramatically increasing the surface area of the small intestine to allow the absorption of food
- releasing enzymes that continue and complete the breakdown/ digestion of food
- absorbing the products of digestion and transporting them into the bloodstream for distribution throughout the body
- acting as a barrier that blocks bacteria, parasites, and toxins from entering the body

Each villus is an independent but intimately related part of the assembly line. It is important to understand that the final stages of digestion, absorption, and transport of nutrients occurs *through*—not between— these tiny, fingerlike projections. When there is inflammation, and a breakdown of the lining of the intestine, the bowel may become permeable, often termed "leaky."

There are *millions* of microscopic villi in each section of the small intestine. Because of its enormous capacity to absorb, parts of it can be damaged with no obvious manifestations or symptoms. But when large sections of the lining are inflamed or destroyed, absorption, enzyme release, transport of nutrients to the body, and the defensive ability of the small intestine is compromised.

Absorption

Once the food components are sufficiently digested (broken down), they are absorbed by different parts of the small intestine.

This is why disease of or infection in one section of the small intestine is often revealed by the malabsorption of specific nutrients. Iron deficiency and metabolic bone disease (e.g., osteoporosis or osteopenia) occur when disease involves the *proximal intestine*, the first two segments of the small intestine. Fat and sugars are absorbed throughout the intestine. Therefore, when one part is diseased, another can compensate and absorb these vital nutrients.

Unless there is a disease process at work, absorption works efficiently and steadily until every usable nutrient in the chyme is absorbed. Nutrients that the body does not need for energy and efficient cellular function are stored for later use—primarily as body fat.

Transport

Once the intestinal wall absorbs the fully digested food, it is transported into the bloodstream and made available to cells throughout the body. Carbohydrates, protein, and fat are transported across the epithelial cell membranes by different mechanisms, with some foods requiring specialized chemical "porters" that literally bind to the components and carry them across the cells of the villi.

Carbohydrates

Carbohydrates supply the body with the fuel it requires for immediate and long-term muscle function and energy. Complex carbohydrates (starches) are usually broken into simple carbs (sugars) in the small intestine. The simple sugars are usually readily transported across the villi into the bloodstream. But some sugars such as lactose or fructose are not absorbed by some people and arrive in the large intestine (colon) mostly undigested. It is these carbohydrates that are thought to cause many of the symptoms of IBS, and their digestive results are often mistaken for gluten intolerance.

Proteins

Proteins are large and complex molecules that are an essential part of every cell, organ, and body system. They are made up of hundreds of amino acids bound together in chemical chains that must be broken down to be used by the body. This is done by enzymes secreted by the pancreas and from the *brush border* (microvilli), which split these chains into smaller and smaller molecules and amino acids that can then be absorbed.

The Problem Protein

Protein is not just found in meat, fish, eggs, and cheese; it is an essential part of many foods. It is the protein portion of wheat—both the gluten and nongluten parts—that gives the small intestine of many people the most trouble. For those with celiac disease, the troublemaker is *gliadin*, the protein portion of wheat and several other grains. It contains one fraction that is not readily digested. So despite all the grinding, churning, mixing, and battering of digestion, some proteins remain intact. Gluten is a major culprit in this scenario.

But scientists are learning that for those with IBS and other gluten sensitivities, it may be the *nongluten* portion of wheat contributing to the problem. (See chapter 11, "Gluten and Nongluten Grains.")

Fat

Fat is one of the major building blocks of the body. It provides long-term energy stores and needed cholesterol. While many people take statins to lower their cholesterol, it is the main component of cell membranes and is needed to maintain the integrity of every cell in the body and to make many hormones.

Mineral and Vitamin Digestion

Specific minerals and vitamins are crucial to body growth, function, and metabolism. Even minor deficiencies disrupt body chemistry.

Vitamins are either water or fat *soluble*. Water-soluble vitamins, the B family and C, move across the watery chyme quite easily either on their own or assisted by special carriers. Fat-soluble vitamins must be *emulsified* to make the trip. Sodium (salt), calcium, iron, water, potassium, and other trace minerals are readily absorbed in different parts of the small intestine, but if the villi are damaged, minerals and vitamins cannot be absorbed.

The Colon (Large Intestine)

Whatever is left of the chyme in the small intestine is then pushed by peristalsis into the colon or large intestine. For many people, this is the part of the digestive tract where painful problems occur.

The digestive process that starts in the mouth culminates in the colon, which is about 6 feet long, shorter than the "small" intestine.

The colon is home to a huge population of bacteria (the microbiota) that have colonized your intestine throughout your lifetime. They feast on everything the small intestine has discarded and digest much of the unused fiber in our diet through fermentation—the bacterial version of chemical conversion. This reduces the chyme into feces and releases folic acid and vitamins B1, B2, B6, B12, and K (the clotting vitamin).

In fact, while the main function of the colon is the absorption of water, approximately 98 percent of the fluids entering from the small intestine—as well as a small but significant percentage of our calories—is actually absorbed in the large intestine. It is the fermentation process that produces carbon dioxide and methane gas, which often translates into flatulence (gas).

As the food is pushed through the colon, the fecal matter becomes more and more concentrated and then stored until it is eliminated through the rectum. The longer it takes to expel feces, the more water is absorbed, making the stool harder and, in turn, more difficult to expel. Diets high in fiber (raw fruits and vegetables, high-fiber cereals) or supplemented with drugstore fiber (e.g., Metamucil or FiberCon) create more fecal bulk that goes largely unabsorbed and creates larger stools.

One of the amazing abilities of the digestive system is its ability to function silently and independently of our brain. We do not need to think about how our food will be digested. The small intestine and much of the colon is controlled by involuntary muscles that work automatically. It is only when things go wrong that we become aware of digestion.

But our brains and extrinsic nerves (facilitated by stress, prunes, and opportunity) play a role in affecting gut muscles. When fecal residue reaches the rectum, we get a signal: We know when there is gas and when there is stool there that needs to be eliminated.

Summary

The digestive system is a wonderfully meshed machine that turns the food we eat into nutrients that support the functions and systems of the body. When all of the interconnected enzymes and secretions, glands and organs, nerve fibers and hormones, muscles and microbes enter and exit as scripted, the play runs smoothly. When any one of these actors is delayed, missing, or becomes overly temperamental, the entire production falters, and sometimes the show cannot go on.

8

The Gut in Disease

When she was good,
She was very good indeed,
But when she was bad she was horrid.
—HENRY WADSWORTH LONGFELLOW,
"THERE WAS A LITTLE GIRL"

Abdominal pain is one of the most common reasons people see a doctor and one of the most difficult symptoms to diagnose. With several notable exceptions (such as a heart attack), most of the pain is caused by problems in the digestive tract. Yet the stages of digestion are so intricately interrelated that disturbances in any one of them—muscles or nerve impulses not working or overworking, enzyme deficiencies, swallowing disorders, infections, reactions to foods or drugs—can result in symptoms and syndromes.

Your digestive system may be falling through the bathroom floor for a number of reasons, but most of the disruptions are not caused by gluten or specific foods. Although randomly eliminating certain foods or drugs may alleviate some symptoms, it is important to *isolate the problem* before you can treat or cure it.

In fact, the underlying conditions that create many of the symptoms attributed to gluten are often diagnosable and treatable without restricting any particular food(s), including gluten. And due to the serious nature of some conditions, it is not just unwise but actually dangerous to ignore them or treat them with diet alone.

Symptoms of GI Disease and Distress

The GI tract is expert in ridding itself of unwanted food and toxins and in letting its "host" know when it is in trouble or simply unhappy. At this point the normally silent workings of digestion raise the volume.

Pain

The truth is rarely pure and never simple.
—OSCAR WILDE

Pain is what drives most people to both the emergency room and the doctor. It is a clear signal of distress, but it is also a complex phenomenon that must be assessed in terms of its location, severity, and duration. Pain is physical—nerves and muscles being pressured, stretched, overstimulated. It is emotional—perceived differently from one individual to another and affected by ongoing or past pain. It is sociocultural—some people are taught to "bear up," and others receive sympathy through expression. Therefore both the triggers of pain and its perception are stimulated and inhibited by many interacting factors that differ from time to time. Some people have bloating and gas pain that they find "like a claw," while others are hardly bothered by it.

The perception of pain in the gut requires perception in the brain.

Nausea and Vomiting

Vomiting is one of the most useful defense mechanisms within the gut. It helps to expel undesirable food from the stomach, including poisons and microbial toxins. It can be triggered by overeating, a reaction to medication, infection, smells or sights, a brain injury, a heart attack, migraines, motion sickness, pregnancy, and other conditions. It is often experienced as a prelude to taking SATs, going onstage in your first major starring role, or meeting your future in-laws.

Vomiting is also a common symptom of gluten ingestion in a usually well-controlled celiac patient.

Diarrhea and Constipation

Most of my meals are very short-term rentals.

(BOB, 49)

I go about once, maybe twice a week. I get my money's worth at a restaurant—the memory and the food linger on.

(SYD, 61)

The word *diarrhea* comes from the ancient Greek meaning "flow through," which characterizes the excessive, frequent, mostly liquid bowel movements of this condition. It can be caused by infections, food poisoning, parasites, medications, lactose intolerance, nerves, fructose, artificial sweeteners, surgery, and a number of digestive disorders. It can be caused by celiac disease and eliminated by a gluten-free diet. Other causes require different treatments.

Patients usually associate diarrhea with large quantities of watery stool. However, physicians define the term as more frequent and/or looser stools. When we ask "Do you have diarrhea?" and the answer is "No, just multiple softer stools," we will write in the chart: "Patient has diarrhea."

Constipation, another common digestive disorder, occurs when bowel movements are less frequent and usually hard. While it is difficult to categorize "normal" for this otherwise normal function, some people go two to three times a day, others that many times a week or month. As explained in the previous chapter, the role of the colon is to absorb water from the stools to keep the body from becoming dehydrated and depleted of necessary minerals. But when feces remain in the large intestine, the water is absorbed out of it, sometimes making it hard and difficult to pass.

Constipation can be caused by reduced intestinal motility (movement) that creates increased storage time, a lack of fiber in the diet, disrupted diet schedules, stress, "holding it in," medications (especially narcotics with codeine), irritable bowel syndrome, and other medical conditions.

People on a strict gluten-free diet often eliminate a fair amount of fiber from their diet in the process and need to replace it to avoid becoming constipated.

Putting Order in the Disorders

The following is a brief description of medically treatable intestinal disorders that all produce symptoms when they attack the 30-foot-long gastrointestinal tract. These can range from cramping and distention to gas, vomiting, diarrhea or constipation, fever, headache, fatigue, and malabsorption (leading to vitamin/mineral deficiencies and neuropathies). These illnesses create similar symptoms, but the diagnoses are as numerous as the tract is long.

Inflammatory Conditions

Inflammation can cause symptoms and signs that are the end product of many different conditions. (See also chapter 15, "Inflammation.")

Inflammatory Bowel Disease
Inflammatory bowel disease (IBD) is the main inflammatory disease of the GI tract. It is a classification that includes Crohn's disease, ulcerative

colitis, collagenous colitis, and lymphocytic colitis. It is diagnosable by radiological imaging and biopsy of the small intestine or colon, and treatable mainly with drugs.

IBD is a serious and potentially life-threatening condition. (For more and evolving information on diet in IBD, see chapter 20.)

Drug-Induced Inflammation

Drugs are an increasingly recognized cause of GI inflammation and distress. Prescribed to treat one condition, they may create another in the process. It is not uncommon for a label to instruct you to "take with food" to prevent stomach upset.

> My doctor prescribed four Advil three times a day for my shoulder pain. Two weeks later I had stomach pain and an ulcer. I should have known better.
>
> (DICK, 70)

A striking example of drug-induced inflammation is familiar to many taking NSAIDs (nonsteroidal anti-inflammatories) or aspirin for arthritis and/or joint pain. Repeated use can inflame the GI tract. Benicar (olmesartan), a drug used to control blood pressure, can cause celiac-like villous atrophy and severe inflammation with associated symptoms, stomach pain, and diarrhea. (See chapter 13, "Drugs.")

We are taking an increasing number of pills to treat everything from pain to fatigue, itching to constipation, weight loss to hair growth. The list of pharmaceuticals used to treat disease today fills 3,250 pages of the *Physicians' Desk Reference*. Each drug has paragraphs of side effects, many of them GI related. The 1,100-page *Handbook of Nonprescription Drugs* published by the American Pharmacists Association is recommended as an "interactive approach to self-care." Again, the number of GI side effects is extensive.

All of these drugs must be absorbed by the GI tract, where they regularly cause significant side effects in the form of inflammation. **Beware of the long-term consequences with any "quick fix."**

(For more, see "Antibiotics" in chapter 9, "The Microbiome," and chapter 13, "Drugs.")

Autoimmune Conditions

There are a number of autoimmune diseases that cause inflammation and disrupt the intestinal tract.

Celiac Disease

Celiac disease is a multisystem disorder where the main target of injury is the small intestine. It inflames and destroys the villi of the small intestine, causing symptoms that are seen throughout the body. (See chapter 17.)

Diabetes

Diabetes attacks the islet cells of the pancreas, creating a lack or deficiency of the hormone insulin that is needed to metabolize glucose, a critical fuel for body function. Type 1, *insulin-dependent diabetes mellitus* (IDDM), destroys the pancreatic islets, requiring permanent insulin injections or an insulin pump. Type 2, *non-insulin-dependent diabetes mellitus* (NIDDM), is not an autoimmune condition, and insulin production is unstable, not absent. (See chapter 23.)

Scleroderma

The word *scleroderma* comes from the Greek *sclero,* meaning "hard," and *derma,* meaning "skin." While hardening and tightening of the skin is one of the most visible manifestations of the disease, the symptoms vary greatly, as do the parts of the body affected. The severity of scleroderma depends on the target as well as the extent of the hardening and tightening.

In people with systemic scleroderma, tissue in the esophagus and gastrointestinal tract (stomach and bowels) can become hard and fibrous, causing them to function less efficiently and affecting digestion. In addition to acid reflux and difficulty swallowing, resulting from damage to the esophagus, some people with scleroderma may also have problems absorbing nutrients if their intestinal muscles lose motility and food is not moving efficiently through the intestines. They can also suffer from diarrhea alternating with constipation. Lack of motility may also contribute to *small intestine bacterial overgrowth* (SIBO).

Since the symptoms of scleroderma are very similar to other autoimmune and GI disorders, it can be mistaken for another condition (GERD or IBS), misdiagnosed, or missed.

Infective Conditions

Infections of the gut (*gastroenteritis*) cause inflammation that disrupts function. Infection is the direct invasion, and inflammation is the reaction. The most common causes of gastroenteritis are:

- Viral infections: rotavirus, Norwalk agent.
- Bacterial infections. These include salmonella, E. coli, yersinia, and shigella. Most of these bacteria are found in food and contaminated water.
- Parasites. These include giardia and cryptosporidia (microscopic parasites found in contaminated water and via human transmission through food and contact) and helminths (flatworms, ringworms, and roundworms that contaminate food, water, and feces).

While most cases of gastroenteritis recover spontaneously or require treatment with antibiotics, antimicrobials, and antiparasitics, many people continue to have intestinal inflammation and symptoms long after the "bugs" are gone. **And the infection can trigger another GI disease.**

There are many people who develop symptoms of celiac disease, IBS, and IBD after bouts of traveler's dysentery, parasites, or another bacterial infection. (See Chapters 17 and 19 for discussions of post-infective celiac disease and IBS.)

Malignant Conditions

GI cancers can occur anywhere in the GI tract from the mouth to the anus, as well as the GI organs (gallbladder, pancreas, liver), and symptoms relate to the location of the malignancy. Colon cancer, the most common GI cancer, is silent until it obstructs or bleeds. Stomach and pancreatic cancer are also silent until they progress to a stage where they impair function, causing symptoms.

At this point, there are links between conditions such as celiac disease, as well as IBD, to an increased incidence of some intestinal cancers and lymphoma. In the absence of celiac disease, no direct link has been made between gluten and malignancy.

Functional Conditions

[IBS] interferes with your life. What is so upsetting is that it is hard to control. I try to eat very plain food in a restaurant. Occasionally you feel great and think: *When is the shoe going to drop?*

(LAURA, 73)

A diseased gut can look normal but not function properly. Functional gastrointestinal disorders (FGIDs), including IBS, are among the most common chronic diseases seen in the general public and affect from 20 to 30 percent of the population at any given time.

They include IBS, gastroparesis, SIBO, GERD, swallowing disorders, and muscle or nervous system problems causing lack of motility or altered function.

Irritable Bowel Syndrome

IBS is a diagnosis of exclusion when symptoms cannot be explained through blood and biopsy/pathology tests or damage to the anatomy of the gut. It is diagnosed by strict criteria. (See chapter 19.)

Gastroparesis

Gastroparesis is a condition where the stomach muscles are not working properly, affecting its ability to empty so that food literally sits there. The backup of food not being propelled down the GI tract into the small intestine can lead to the characteristic feeling of fullness before finishing a meal, occasional overgrowth of bacteria in the small intestine, the hardening of undigested food in the stomach (which can obstruct its passage into the small intestine), and blood sugar fluctuations. Gastroparesis may contribute to or aggravate GERD, especially at night.

The causes of gastroparesis are not fully known, but uncontrolled diabetes, damage to the nerves in the stomach or even the vagus nerve (which regulates chemical levels in the digestive system that signal the stomach to empty), scleroderma, and certain drugs such as opiates may cause or contribute to the condition. It has also been proposed that damage to the nerves controlling involuntary functions—such as stomach emptying—occurs.

The management of gastroparesis is primarily dietary, with medications prescribed when necessary. Patients are directed to avoid foods that delay gastric emptying, such as fatty foods, red meat, and high-fiber foods. Small, more frequent meals and soft and/or liquid foods also improve emptying.

Gastroparesis is common in celiac disease and may improve with a gluten-free diet.

Small Intestinal Bacterial Overgrowth

The entire GI tract is lined with bacteria. (See chapter 9, "The Microbiome.") The number as well as the composition of these bacteria differs from the small intestine to the colon, with the majority of our microbiota in the large intestine. SIBO occurs when bacteria that are normally found in the colon flourish in the small intestine.

It can occur when gut motility (movement) is impaired and bacteria linger in the small intestine and multiply, or when the small intestine is obstructed and food cannot move along. Diverticula (small sacs protruding from the intestinal wall) can also allow bacteria to accumulate and multiply within them.

Like many of the functional conditions of the GI tract, SIBO can cause flatulence, bloating, constipation, diarrhea, and pain. When SIBO is severe or goes undiagnosed, bacteria can interfere with digestion and cause vitamin and mineral deficiencies and weight loss. The resulting inflammation can also produce fatigue. **SIBO is a condition that is often mistaken for gluten sensitivity or intolerance.**

It can be diagnosed with a hydrogen breath test (see chapter 6, "Testing") or sampling of intestinal fluid.

SIBO is treated with antibiotics and probiotics or a combination of both. While most doctors will not keep patients on repeated courses of antibiotics due to long-term side effects, many do not have the same reluctance to recommend prolonged probiotic use. (See chapter 5, "Supplements and Probiotics.") Long-term studies comparing antibiotics, probiotics, and combinations of antibiotics and probiotics are needed.

Gastroesophageal Reflux Disease

I always had this very dramatic cough. In the winter I would get these scary coughs that were so deep, that wouldn't stop and wouldn't go away. About eight years ago, we were on vacation, and I went to a doctor and they put me on antibiotics, but the cough wouldn't go away. When I came back I went to a pulmonologist. He started doing breathing tests on me and then said I had asthma. So he put me on all types of asthma meds. It didn't really do very much, and I just didn't question it. I'm one who doesn't like to question authority.

Fortunately, I had a doctor friend who said, "I really wish you'd see someone else, because I think it has something to do with your esophagus, your vocal cords." I finally got to a doctor who deals with the nose down to the stomach, very unusual. She gave me all kinds of tests and diagnosed me as having silent reflux. I don't feel it. When I had reflux I coughed. Coughing was the only symptom. No sore throat.

She put me on a very, very restrictive food program for six months, and when it didn't help, she recommended a fundoplication [surgery that strengthens the valve between the stomach and the esophagus so acid does not back up]. So that was really amazingly helpful.

After a couple of years I started coughing again. So, I went on medication and on a very low pH diet again. I was on the diet more than a year, and it helped solve the issue.

I call it the "elevator syndrome." Someone says, "You should see someone for your chest," and you get on the elevator and you get off on the floor with all the chest doctors and they diagnose you with a chest issue. But if you'd gotten off two floors down and happen to go to a gastroenterologist, they might give you a diagnosis based on a stomach or gut issue. It all depends on the floor you get off on.

(LYNDSEY, 61)

GERD occurs when stomach acid or the contents of the stomach flow back into the esophagus. The reflux (meaning to return or flow back) irritates the lining of the esophagus, causing burning, chest pain, cough, hoarseness, a sore throat, or *globus* (the sensation of a lump in the throat). Anyone who has ever suffered from GERD will tell you that the sour liquid filled with stomach acid seriously irritates the unprotected lining of the throat.

GERD can be caused by a number of physical, dietary, and lifestyle issues. They include a weakness in the sphincter that closes the esophageal opening (food is only supposed to go down the GI tract, not back up), a *hiatal hernia,* and certain foods. Pregnancy and obesity may also contribute to the problem.

GERD is treated with changes to diet, eating times (eating right before lying down to sleep can make the transit of food downward from the stomach more difficult), weight loss, and other lifestyle changes. Various over-the-counter (OTC) and prescription drugs are also recommended for some patients. The amount of shelf space devoted to OTC remedies for reflux testifies to the prevalence of the condition.

The GERD diet does not usually restrict gluten, but patients with celiac disease can also suffer from the condition. Of those people who are tested for GERD we have found about 10 percent are diagnosed with celiac disease. For these patients, the gluten-free diet relieves the symptoms, and they are able to stop taking prescribed medications. Reflux can therefore be a manifestation of celiac disease.

Pregnancy Disruptions

I think I burped my baby out.

(RIANNE, 35)

Many women have jokingly referred to pregnancy as a nine-month series of GI disruptions. In fact, much of the GI tract and its related organs are rearranged and compressed as the fetus grows. This can alter bowel, digestive, and urinary function, causing reflux, gastroparesis, nausea, gas, and bloating. Most of these are triggered by hormonal changes, but some may be a function of the increased pressure on the GI tract. Problems are compounded because women cannot take the usual medications to treat these conditions.

Pregnancy can also make a pre-existing GI condition worse—studies have documented an increased flare-up of IBD in the first trimester of pregnancy and postpartum. (For more, see chapter 9, "The Microbiome.")

Infiltrative Conditions

Diseases such as ulcers and *collagenous sprue* cause lesions or scars that penetrate the mucosal lining of the GI tract. While ulcers are neither caused by gluten ingestion nor cured by its removal from the diet, collagenous sprue does have an interesting relation to gluten.

Ulcers

Peptic ulcers are defects in the surface layer or mucous lining of the GI tract. They occur mainly in the stomach and the duodenum but can appear anywhere. Occasionally they may be deep and extend through the entire bowel wall, perforating the bowel.

The stomach and duodenum come into constant contact with gastric acid and enzymes, yet are not usually damaged by acid resulting in ulcers. It used to be believed that ulcers were a result of stress or acid and exacerbated by certain foods (e.g., alcohol, caffeine, tobacco, excess roughage, rich and fatty foods). However, Drs. Barry Marshall and J. Robin Warren won the Nobel Prize for their "remarkable and unexpected discovery" that ulceration of the stomach or duodenum—peptic ulcer disease—is the result of an infection of the stomach caused by *Helicobacter pylori*. Smoking and the overuse of NSAIDs (ibuprofen, naproxen, Aleve) and aspirin are the only other known causes of peptic ulcers. Ulcers lower in the GI tract are not acid or *H. pylori* related.

Interestingly, some studies show that older adults are more likely to develop ulcers, and this may in fact be a result of their increased use of aspirin and NSAIDs to control arthritis pain.

Fortunately, peptic ulcers are relatively easy to treat with antibiotics and other drugs, such as proton pump inhibitors, which reduce the amount of acid produced by the stomach. Because of the danger of bleeding and the resulting anemia and/or stomach cancer, ulcers should be diagnosed and monitored by your doctor.

Collagenous Sprue

Collagenous sprue is a lesion within the small intestine that occurs in those with villous atrophy. It is so named because of a band of collagen (scar tissue) that forms right under the epithelial cells lining the intestine. Its symptoms mimic many other GI diseases, and it is typically associated with severe malabsorption and diarrhea. It can be caused by any kind of sprue—tropical, celiac, or drug-induced.

Celiac disease that does not normalize on a gluten-free diet is often called "refractory sprue" (type 1 and type 2) and can develop into collagenous sprue. This is treated with a combination of a gluten-free diet, steroids, or other immunosuppressants.

Miscellaneous Disorders of the Normal Gut

Lactose Intolerance

Lactose intolerance is caused by a lack of the enzyme (*lactase*) that digests lactose, the sugar found in milk and milk products. There are two types of lactose intolerance—primary, which is genetic, and secondary, which is caused by the destruction of the microvilli of the small intestine that produce lactase (see chapter 7, "The Normal Gut and Digestion"). Secondary lactose intolerance occurs in celiac disease and many other conditions when inflammation "sears" and destroys the microvilli. It usually resolves when the underlying condition is treated and cured.

When undigested lactose arrives in the colon and is fermented by the bacteria—which thrive on this sugar—it then causes the bloating, gas, and diarrhea common to sufferers of lactose intolerance.

Genetic lactose intolerance is treated by the avoidance of milk products and the use of lactase supplements when ice cream and pizza beckon. Secondary lactose intolerance is treated by the resolution of the underlying condition causing the villous atrophy.

Summary

- A diseased gut sends signals in the form of symptoms, and interpreting them can be confusing. Symptoms are complex, and the same symptoms can underlie different problems with different treatments.

- Symptoms can evolve. Bacterial and parasitic infections in the GI tract can trigger other conditions. This is often the reason that symptoms do not resolve but progress into another problem.

- GI problems fall into four basic categories. They can be caused by inflammatory conditions, malignancies, functional, and/or infiltrative issues. Putting yourself on a gluten-free diet will not necessarily resolve the underlying problem and may delay a proper diagnosis and cure.

- Do not give in to the temptation to self-diagnose and blame the food you eat for GI symptoms.

- It is critical to isolate, test, and then treat.

9

The Microbiome

Exploring the unknown requires tolerating uncertainty.
—BRIAN GREENE, THEORETICAL PHYSICIST

If you don't like bacteria, you're on the wrong
planet. This is the planet of the bacteria.
—CRAIG VENTER, BIOTECHNOLOGIST,
BIOCHEMIST, AND GENETICIST

The human body is home to trillions of tiny organisms that vastly out-number the cells in the body and affect our overall health. In fact, there are approximately 10 trillion cells in the human body and 100 trillion living microorganisms. These are the bacteria, viruses, fungi, and yeast that compose the microbiota.* They line all the surfaces of the body and live in the GI tract from mouth to anus as well as the skin, nose, teeth, and ears, and the male and female sexual organs.

The human body is their home, and they have evolved distinct "personalities" amenable to their particular living arrangements. There is even seasonal variability in our skin microbiota. But it is in the gut that most of them exist and flourish. Some thrive in the acidity of the stomach, others

---

* The term *microbiota* encompasses the trillions of microbes living in and on the human body; the term *microbiome* technically means the collective genome of the microbiota. They are often used interchangeably.

in the dark and wet large intestine. Microbiota are integral to the digestive process and the constant internal dialogue between the immune, metabolic, and nervous systems. They play a crucial role in human development and health, and are routinely affected by everything we put in our mouths.

They are a fulcrum of metabolism, releasing nutrients from foods that would be otherwise indigestible, and making B vitamins and vitamin K. They create a constant state of inflammation and immune regulation so that we do not identify all proteins as foreign and can also tolerate food products. In fact, the microbiome trains our immune system very early in life. They are part of the "tasting" system that samples foreign proteins and pathogens entering the gut, determining if they are safe or harmful, and then instructing the immune system.

These various organisms are often referred to as commensal bacteria, which derives from the Latin *com* (in association) and *mensal* (at the table or meal). We quite literally "eat at the same table" with our microbiotic family since the food we eat is their main source of energy. And everything we ingest plays a role in dictating which will thrive and which will perish.

Researchers now know that the relationship we have with our microbiome can best be described as one of *amphibiosis*—as Martin Blaser, M.D., explains in his book *Missing Microbes*[*]—it is symbiotic (mutually dependent) or parasitic depending on context. Our microbiome works with and against us at any given time—and often simultaneously.

Everyone's microbiome is his or her own personal jar of multicolored jelly beans that gets shaken and rearranged, eaten, and replaced regularly. There are shifts in both the diversity and the pattern of each individual's bacterial makeup over time as well as within different cultures around the world.

Disruption in the microbiome is known as *dysbiosis* (*dys*—abnormal, impaired; *biosis*—mode of life), an imbalance in the microbiota, and this has different effects on the body and our health. There is the possibility that the manipulation of the microbiome may be a link between risk fac-

---

* *Missing Microbes*, Martin J. Blaser, M.D., Henry Holt and Co., 2014, p. 99.

tors and development of many disorders ranging from diabetes to obesity. Intestinal dysbiosis has been associated with celiac disease, but whether the alterations in the microbiome are cause or consequence of the disease is unknown.

It is also possible that a specific genetic makeup may influence the composition of the first gut colonizers and could contribute to determining your risk for certain diseases. This is being studied in a number of neurological conditions and mood disorders as well as the gut.

Diet can also alter the composition of your flora and fauna. People on a vegan or vegetarian or very restricted diet can change the composition of their fecal microbiota. Yet there is no scientific proof as to the effect of this alteration and whether the microbiota returns to their "normal" once the diet changes. The diet can affect the composition, but not permanently. (Unless it is your permanent diet.)

We are currently studying the effects of a gluten-free diet on both celiac and gluten-sensitive volunteers to determine if it can change their microbiome.

The hot topic for scientists today is what this all means—the creation, growth, composition, mechanisms, and roles of the microbiome. Currently, almost any disease process that is looked at may be associated with alterations in the microbiome, and we may be applying "treatments" where they are unnecessary and/or harmful. There are many unanswered questions surrounding the rush to manipulate the microbiome with probiotics and a daily infusion of yogurt.

Where Does the Microbiome Come From?

You can choose your friends, but not your relatives.
—ANONYMOUS

Our microbiota come to us both vertically and horizontally—that is, from our genes and constantly from our environment. We initially acquire our microbiome from our mother, but every child is also a product of the parental genes.

Bacteria line the birth canal and are introduced into the baby during childbirth. Exposure continues through suckling, licking, touching, and kissing the baby. Long before blenders, Beech-Nut, and Gerber, parents used to chew baby's food, and even now, mothers often use their saliva to wipe a smear of dirt from a child's mouth or face. The antibodies that are transferred from mother to child across the placenta and through breast-feeding are protective against infections and possibly dietary anti-gens. Everyone and everything a baby touches or consumes also feeds its microbiome. By the age of 3, the child's microbiome resembles that of an adult and stabilizes.

The adult microbiome continues to incorporate this horizontal and vertical input that changes as we age through the drugs we take; the food, vitamins, and supplements we ingest; the people we kiss and touch; the places we travel to; and the diseases we acquire. This ever-evolving, dynamic, and complex ecosystem differs not only from individual to individual but in the same person over time. Microbiota also differ from country to country depending on what you eat and where you live, and differ when you are sick.

More important, our microbiome has its own genetic component that is 100 times more complex than the human genome.

The 21st-Century Microbiome

The contemporary Western world has evolved—now we are all washing our hands, giving birth to babies in hospitals and not on the kitchen table, sterilizing baby bottles and nipples, and maintaining a level of cleanliness not seen either in our earlier human history or even in other parts of the world. And it is becoming clear that this emphasis on cleanliness has repercussions. (See chapter 3, "The Hygiene Hypothesis.") We are also taking various antibiotics—"drugs that kill bugs"—that change the composition of our microbiome.

While there is no one "healthy" microbiome, there is little doubt that 21st-century life has—and is—altering our intestinal ecosystem with ramifications for our health. When the microbiome is disrupted it upsets the entire body—slowly or rapidly depending on the degree of dysbiosis. While the active microorganisms within us may offer new keys to GI health and repair, we first must try to ascertain what comes first—the disease or the dysbiosis. That is, do changes in the microbiome initiate a disease, or are they a result of it? Quite possibly, they co-exist in an elaborate dance where genes, germs, and environment take turns leading.

Why Is It Important?

If we knew what it was we were doing, it would
not be called research, would it?
—ALBERT EINSTEIN

Since the microbiome is extremely diverse, even in healthy people, and most diseases have various subtypes and manifestations, it is very difficult to pinpoint a direct cause-and-effect relation between the microbiome and specific diseases. This complex and unpredictable system thrives because of its ability to respond so rapidly to change. We must attempt to decode the dialogue between the microbiome and the immune system of the body before we can understand its messages.

The following are a number of factors that scientists have isolated as affecting the microbiome. Keep in mind that the consequences of these changes are unclear.

Pregnancy and the Microbiome

While some bacteria may enter the child via the placenta in utero, the bulk of the newborn's microbiome is colonized during birth when the microbes in the mother's vagina populate the child's body. Thus, there is a biological cost to an elective Caesarean section (as opposed to an emergency C-section when the child has already descended into the birth canal) for the newborn. As Martin Blaser, M.D., notes in *Missing Microbes,* the "founding populations of microbes found on C-section infants are not those selected by hundreds of thousands of years of human evolution or even longer." He asks, "What if those first microbial residents provide signals that critically interact with cells in the rapidly developing baby's body?" Studies have shown a connection between C-section babies, obesity, and celiac disease, as well as other disorders. Yet other studies have questioned the link.

There are interesting links between the colonization of the infant microbiome and various diseases and disorders, but the effect of genetics and infant environment leave much unanswered. We often hear remarks like "stomach issues run in our family." Certain diseases—e.g., celiac disease, Crohn's disease—have a genetic basis but also environmental triggers. This raises the intriguing issue of whether the mother's dysbiosis is passed genetically, acquired later or during pregnancy, and what effect, if any, it has on the newborn.

The jury is still out on this.

Antibiotics and the Microbiome

If we have coevolved with our microbiome, what happens when we take multiple courses of antibiotics that kill bacteria—both good and bad, either permanently or only at times—rearranging our intestinal flora or impacting our immune systems? Does that impact give certain conditions a chance to flourish or occur?

The average child in the U.S. has taken between three and four courses of antibiotics before his/her third birthday, when a child's microbiome is still plastic. In 2013, a nationwide study showed that half of all children in many Western countries receive antibiotics at least once a year. Allergies, celiac disease, autoimmune diseases, obesity, and autism diagnoses have mushroomed in the past decade. Some scientists believe antibiotics may be responsible for the rise in these and other conditions because of their effect on the microbiome and the resonating effect this has on the immune system.

Antibiotics also have a direct effect on the gut that can be easily demonstrated. Bacteria in the colon make vitamin K, which helps to clot our blood and stop excessive bleeding (see chapter 7, "Digestion"). But if you are taking antibiotics that kill the bacteria making vitamin K and you are also taking a blood thinner, such as Coumadin, you can get massively high levels of anticoagulation. This can be a huge problem.

Most of the many species of microorganisms in the digestive tract are helpful under normal circumstances. But when something upsets the balance of these organisms, an otherwise harmless bacteria can grow out of control and create huge problems. An example of this is a bacterium called *Clostridium difficile*, or *C. diff.* When illness and/or different drugs wipe out competing bacteria, this usually benign organism overgrows the compromised intestine, releases toxins that attack the lining of the intestines, and causes severe colitis and diarrhea and occasionally death.

The disturbance of normal healthy bacteria by antibiotics, acid suppression and age may provide *C. difficile* an opportunity to overrun the intestinal microbiome. It is carried in feces and acquired from contaminated surfaces including hands and equipment. In a healthy person's gut, it is contained by other thriving bacteria. Outbreaks therefore are often found in settings with compromised patients, such as hospitals and nursing homes. (See "Bugs as Drugs" later in this chapter and in chapter 30.)

It is clear that a disturbed microbiome reduces the body's ability to respond to and tolerate the many things we ingest.

Microbiome and Food Allergies

There has been a large rise in childhood food allergies over the past decades. Research from animal studies indicates that a microbiome diminished and/or changed by antibiotics may be a factor in this increase in allergic and immune responses.

In a recent study, mice given antibiotics early in life were far more susceptible to peanut sensitization, a model of human peanut allergy. When the mice were fed a solution containing *Clostridia,* a common gut bacterium, the sensitization disappeared. When given *Bacteroides,* another kind of common and healthy bacteria, the same effect was not found. The researchers determined that *Clostridia* helped to "maintain the integrity of the [intestinal] barrier," which kept peanut proteins that can cause allergic reactions out of the bloodstream. While these researchers have concluded that it may be possible to manipulate the microbiota as allergy therapy, all of this needs testing in humans.

This and other research "opens up new territory," Blaser says. It "extends the frontier of how the microbiome is involved" in immune responses and the roles played by specific bacteria.

Research studies suggest that factors that alter the microbiome increase the risk of developing celiac disease. Most of the risk factors for celiac disease—elective Caesarean, gastrointestinal infections, antibiotic or proton pump inhibitor use—could also be interpreted as modulators of the microbiome. Some studies show that children with a genetic risk for celiac disease have different microbiota compared to other children.

Obesity and the Microbiome

There are several "nonintuitive" disruptions to the microbiome that are attracting scientific interest, such as obesity theories. Researchers have found more diversity in the microbiome of leaner people. This has raised the question of whether antibiotics contribute to the development of obesity, since they kill bacteria. Several hypotheses are suggesting manipulating the microbiome to treat obesity and metabolic disorders.

There are a number of mechanisms by which intestinal bacteria may promote obesity. Some studies demonstrate that certain bacteria improve the absorption of nutrients in the small intestine—possibly promoting weight gain.

Other studies point a finger at the ability of microbes to increase inflammation. Since intestinal inflammation has been seen as a condition preceding obesity and metabolic disease, and this can be altered by dietary changes of the gut microbiota, it is possible that dietary intervention can be designed to combat these disorders.

Finally, the levels of certain families of bacteria differ in obese and lean people, which lends support to the theory of a microbial link in obesity. But it is still unknown whether people are genetically prone to lower levels of specific classes of bacteria, making them prone to obesity.

In mouse studies, microbiota from obese patients transferred obesity to the mice, leading to the assumption that microbiota can be causative and transmissible.

We have learned from farmers that giving antibiotics to farm animals makes them grow fatter and faster. With studies showing that antibiotics change the microbiota, we must question the antibiotics that are now in our meat and our milk and the consequences of this approach on us and our children.

It is important to know that these theories are controversial, but it is clear that what we ingest plays a major role in the composition of the microbiota and therefore its function. Dietary strategies targeting the microbes in our gut may be a possible tool to control metabolic disorders and obesity. Research trials using diets, probiotics, prebiotics, or a combination are in very early stages. We need to understand the complex interactions between our genes, our germs, and everything we ingest before a treatment strategy can be determined.

Autism Spectrum Disorder and the Microbiome

It has been hypothesized that changes in the gut microbiota play a role in the development of autism. We will explore some of the proposed mechanisms linking such changes to neurological development, immune function, and behavior in chapter 26, "Autism."

The Microbiome and the Brain—
Can Bacteria Change Behavior?

The link between our microbiota and our brains is another part of the new frontier. It has been studied mainly in mice, with intriguing results. Through them scientists have shown that microbiota are not only important to healthy metabolism and brain function, but that the gut-brain communication pathways include the enteric nervous system (see chapter 10, "The 'Second Brain'"), and that the development of gut microbiota may influence the wiring of circuits that affect stress and impact mood and behavior. Many of these studies involve germ-free mice with controlled introduction of antibiotics, bacteria, and foods. Caution is required since the mouse intestinal tract is not a substitute for the human. But researchers have "humanized" mice by inserting human genes associated with different diseases into them, and this is an opportunity to study the relationship between specific genes and diseases as well as the effect of drugs and dysbiosis in various conditions.

Many people consider chocolate and coffee the ultimate "mood foods"—capable of calming frazzled nerves and restoring energy. These foods actually contain chemicals that stimulate the brain. Researchers in Canada are now examining the influence of food on the composition and activity of our intestinal bacteria and whether this can influence brain function and mood. They have shown that specific probiotic mixtures can restore normal feeding behavior in mice whose patterns had become distorted after a stomach infection. These researchers are now investigating a specific probiotic for IBS and its effect on GI as well as psychiatric symptoms. They caution that the mouse research attempting to alter behavior by modifying bacteria in the gut cannot be translated to humans at this point.

Bugs as Drugs

Before the discovery and routine use of antibiotics in the 20th century, elixirs and tinctures of herbs and plants as well as actual bugs were routinely used to treat infections and various illnesses. The line between food, plants, worms, and medicine was thin. Today, antimicrobials—which include antibacterials, antivirals, antifungals, and antiparasitics—target every organism in our microbiotic ecosystem. Unfortunately, designed for adaptation and experienced over millions of years in survival techniques, bacteria and viruses have developed resistance to many of these drugs and found ways to elude them.

Because antimicrobial resistance is now a major health issue, researchers are using bacteria, "bugs," and viruses themselves to fight disease. They are also using the ability to decode the genome to find new treatments to circumvent the growing crisis of drug resistance. Maggots, leeches, and herbal remedies are making a comeback as well.

Fecal transplants have recently been approved as therapy for resistant and recurrent *C. difficile* infection, and are under investigation for a host of other conditions. Stool, frequently from a relative or other healthy donor, is examined for different pathogens, mixed with a saline solution, and introduced into the patient's intestines via enemas or during a colonoscopy and/or upper endoscopy. The intent is to replace the "good bacteria" that has been killed by illness, drugs, or the *C. difficile* in order to restore the missing flora and suppress the *C. diff* that has overrun the intestines.

One researcher noted that "the intestinal flora is a promising new frontier for scientists and health care professionals alike." The question is not only whether the newly introduced outsider will stay but what effect he will have on the neighborhood.

How Constant Is the Microbiome?

If you alter the microbiome by changing your diet or taking pro- or prebiotics, what are the short- and long-term effects? This is a key question and the focus of most of the current research. Studies have shown that if you give antibiotics to a very young child, the microbiota will permanently change. When they are given later, the composition returns to what it was. But science is not at a point in its understanding of the microbiome to know what the short- and/or long-term effects are of these changes.

There is also the question of the safety of probiotics. Under what conditions are they made, and where? Are they viable? Can you trust the label? The recent death of a child due to contaminated probiotics is unacceptable. (See chapter 5, "Supplements and Probiotics.")

Summary

- The intestinal microbiome is an immense ecosystem within our body. It orchestrates and maintains stability in the digestive and immune systems by constantly responding to what we ingest and changes in external conditions.

- The microbiome is populated both vertically, i.e., genetically and from our mother during birth, and horizontally, by everything we eat, touch, and breathe. Its composition is therefore continually changing and rearranging.

- It is active in metabolism by helping to digest food that is otherwise indigestible and releasing vitamins and minerals.

- Everyone's microbiome is different and varies in any individual over time and circumstances. It changes with age, diet, and disease.

- The microbiome is instrumental in controlling inflammation in the gut—in effect, turning the gas up or down. Our ability to react to pathogens and intestinal disease depends on this microbiotic hand on the intestinal "oven."

- Chronic inflammation and/or dysbiosis can bring about a series of events that lead to altered bowel function, intestinal diseases such as IBS, and, it is hypothesized, various autoimmune diseases including IBD, celiac disease, autism spectrum disorder, type 1 diabetes, and obesity.

- If bacteria in the gut strays from its usual home, it can cause both systemic as well as gut diseases.

- Sometimes "good" bacteria is killed off by antibiotics or other drugs, and "bad" bacteria overruns the system, creating dysbiosis, or disruptions in the microbiota.

- It may be possible to modify the intestinal microbiota by diet, prebiotics, probiotics, or fecal transplant of donor stool. But little is known about the best types of interventions, the degree of resistance to a particular therapy, or the long-term effect of any therapy.

- Food and drugs, such as antibiotics, affect and alter the micro-organisms in the gut. Conversely, it is also possible that any one person's microbiota may also affect the response to certain foods (such as gluten) and the efficacy or toxicity of drugs he or she takes. This requires more research on both genes and germs to determine the role of each microbial species.
- The microbiome is the new frontier in GI health. While it appears to offer tantalizing answers to many things affecting the body, the truth is proving to be as elusive as the many microscopic organisms eating at our table.

10

The "Second Brain" in the Gut

. . . who wears his wit in his belly, and his guts in his head . . .
—SHAKESPEARE, *TROILUS AND CRESSIDA*

In every body, the brain is king. Its writ is law. At the top of the bowel, the rule of the king is acknowledged, but as one descends deeper and deeper into the depths of the gut, the rule of the king weakens. A new order emerges: that of the second brain.
—MICHAEL D. GERSHON, M.D., *THE SECOND BRAIN*

The belly rules the mind.
—SPANISH PROVERB

Digestion has evolved over millions of years into a highly efficient work-horse that enables us to digest food without conscious thought—freeing us for evolutionarily desirable activities like hunting, mating, and escaping danger and the modern equivalents of working, shopping, and texting. It is only when this system raises itself to the level of consciousness and sends SOS messages—cramps, diarrhea, heartburn—that we become consciously aware of its workings.

The independent nature of our gut and the interactions between the brain and the gut have been well known for many centuries. They are an important aspect of normal GI function and to the way we think and feel. Treating GI symptoms requires an understanding and appreciation of our "second brain."

I feel as if I have two brains—one in my gut and one in my head.

(GLEN, 50)

My gut was always sensitive to emotional things. When I was in a stressful situation I would get diarrhea. Something terrible would happen, and that would be the trigger.

(CARLA, 40, IBS)

Nervous System 101

In simplest terms, the nervous system consists of two main branches that work together to control all bodily functions. It is divided into the central nervous system (CNS), consisting of the brain and spinal cord, and the peripheral nervous system (PNS), which sends nerve fibers to and from the brain and spinal cord to the rest of the body. The CNS is the "top dog," and the PNS carries out orders and reports back with constant updates on bodily status. The autonomic nervous system (ANS) is a branch of the PNS and controls functions in the body that work independently of conscious control and awareness, e.g., sweating, heartbeat, and digestion.

The enteric nervous system (ENS) is the intrinsic (located within) division of the ANS that governs the functions of the gut—it does not need constant orders from the brain/spinal cord to function, although it reports back and stays in constant communication with the central nervous system. If you take a piece of bowel and isolate it, it has movement. It contracts automatically because there are local nervous connections within it to the intestinal muscles that act independently.

Thus, while all of the nervous system is interconnected and constantly engaged in cross-talk, the enteric nervous system is a "second brain" in the body.

The Enteric Nervous System

There are 100 million nerve cells in the small intestine, roughly equivalent to the number in the spinal cord. It is the largest and most complex division of the PNS and ANS, and consists of numerous different types of neurons. They monitor and control both the "automatic" aspects of digestion—which require no conscious thought to function—and the very real functional and nervous conditions it is involved in.

There are different types of nerve cells embedded within the walls of the GI tract, and each has anatomical features that reflect the cells' functions. An explanation of these different cells is beyond the scope of this book, but it is important to know that they have control over the stimulation and/or inhibition of motor activities and secretions in the bowel.

You might think of the ENS as an integrated circuit board—the "motherboard" of the system—that is involved in all aspects of intestinal function. It integrates GI motility/movement, the exchange of fluids across the mucosal surface of the intestine, blood flow, and the secretion of gut hormones. The ENS controls, coordinates, and impacts food regulation, digestion, and absorption as well as the development and perception of symptoms through its many sensory mechanisms. It is an integral and crucial component of the nervous system but capable of self-government as well as rebellion.

It acts independently, can learn and respond to emotions, and "remembers" in order to produce "gut" feelings.

> I had the most outrageous pain in my lower abdomen—a take-your-breath-away, knifelike pain.
>
> (MARION, 68)

> I have an iron-man belly; nothing I eat or do affects it!
>
> (MARSHAL, 65)

While the ENS normally runs silent and deep like a submarine, when it is altered in disease, it "surfaces," breaks radio silence, and rapidly expresses its distress. It is also capable of shooting ballistic pain missiles. This comes as no surprise to the 30 percent of all patients who visit doctors yearly for GI complaints. They have no trouble understanding that the ENS is also a sensory organ. But its "senses" are multilayered.

The GI Tract as Sensory Organ

In order to protect itself from the outside world, the GI tract must be able to mount appropriate defenses against pathogens and other harmful substances. At the same time, it must be open and permeable to nutrients. It integrates these two responses by a multifaceted detection system that senses the outside environment and then reacts appropriately. It identifies friend from foe and acts on that knowledge. It can reject foods through objectionable taste, vomiting, diarrhea, or any combination of these symptoms. This occurs through a very complex system of nerve and immune cells that line the tract and trigger responses such as nausea, vomiting, and pain. Vomiting and diarrhea can be rapid responses if toxic substances are ingested in sufficient quantities.

But the sensors can malfunction and initiate reactions that are responsible for many digestive problems—as many people with IBS will attest. As Michael Gershon, M.D. (an expert in the growing field of neurogastroenterology), notes in his book *The Second Brain,* "Few things are more distressing than an inefficient gut with feeling. And, since the enteric nervous system can function on its own, it must be considered possible that the brain in the bowel may have its own psychoneuroses."

Many of the patients we interviewed complain that doctors tell them "It's all in your head" and prescribe a psychotropic. Their response to that is a vigorous "I am not depressed!" But it is becoming increasingly clear that many of these drugs are actually "gut-otropics"—therapies aimed at the "second brain" in the gut. A reversal in thinking on this subject may be an important answer to treating functional bowel disease.

While our understanding of the integrated responses of the gut to the sensory information it receives is growing, it is only in the early stages of developing therapeutic agents and dietary approaches that target specific gut receptors. One such receptor, serotonin, is receiving increased attention as both "sword and shield." If we can "sculpt" the ENS, we may be able to block the responses that lead to malfunctions in the GI tract and echo throughout the body.

The Molecular Busybody

Nerves act by releasing neurotransmitters, molecules that stimulate or inhibit a target receptor. These nervous impulses, like electrical transmission, release a host of different chemicals that initiate the "on" or "off" switch. One of the key chemicals in this scenario is serotonin.

What Is a Brain Chemical Doing in the Gut?

Serotonin was always considered a brain chemical—a neurotransmitter—mainly because it is targeted as a therapy for depression. But, in fact, 95 percent of the serotonin in your body can be found in your gut.

Serotonin is much more than a mood elevator. It has multiple functions—it is a "busybody" because its nose is into everything and everybody's business, and in particular it does this in the GI tract.

Serotonin has a number of important functions:

- It is critical in development, a growth factor.
- It is a hormone that moves from the gut into the bloodstream and regulates bone development.
- It regulates movement in the intestines. In other words, *too little* serotonin can contribute to constipation (or slow transit time). *Too much* serotonin can contribute to diarrhea (or fast transit time).

- It is a defensive molecule. The cells making serotonin have sensors that can detect bacteria. This causes serotonin to be released and can activate the immune system and start inflammation. This serves to warn the body of infection. If this malfunctions, it can lead to unwanted inflammation. But in reality, these antithetical functions are actually synergistic and, as Dr. Gershon notes, "allow the gut to have its inflammation and survive it too."

- It is a paracrine hormone (acting only in the vicinity of the gland secreting it) that stimulates peristalsis, movement in the gut that propels food down the GI tract.

- It is a neurotransmitter in the ENS involved in many nerve functions.

The role of serotonin in the GI tract is an emerging area of study. It may have a central role in GI function and the development of disease. It is important to gastrointestinal motility, intestinal neurogenesis, mucosal growth/maintenance, intestinal inflammation, and bone growth. Serotonin receptors are being actively studied as therapeutic targets to treat IBS, obesity, and type 2 diabetes, and as a potential sculptor of the ENS. Its true role has yet to be determined.

Can We Train or "Sculpt" the ENS?

Altering the activities of serotonin is being actively studied to produce long-lasting changes in the ENS. Since IBS and other GI conditions often begin in childhood, it is hoped that by "sculpting" the development of neurons, the pathways for and development of various psychological or infectious/inflammatory reactions could be influenced.

Work on the ENS has many diagnostic and study challenges, since it is difficult to test intestinal nervous tissue. Most of the current studies are on mice, many with human gene mutations.

Serotonin has become part of the arsenal of antidepressants such as tricyclic antidepressants and selective serotonin reuptake inhibitors (SSRIs) that are effective in the treatment of both *affective* (mood) and GI disorders. These drugs treat the active part of the gut that talks to the brain quieting the GI tract and the pain. It also quiets the part of the brain making the gut upset.

When taking serotonin, you are treating the "second brain" in the gut.

> *It's not "all in your head"—a great deal is in your gut.*
> —MICHAEL GERSHON, M.D.

Summary

- The gut has a mind of its own—the enteric nervous system. The ENS is one of the most intriguing parts of the brain-gut complex and involved in and/or responsible for many of the symptoms of GI disease and malfunction.
- The ENS is an efficient computing center that sends nerve, immunological, and hormonal messages throughout the GI tract and cross-talk to other parts of the body.
- The receptors in the gut think, feel, and stimulate responses and/or inhibit them—often simultaneously. They are the targets of much research. Training or "sculpting" them may enable scientists to prevent as well as treat GI malfunction and conditions.
- When we evaluate and treat GI conditions, we must also acknowledge and treat this ruler of "the lower kingdom."

PART III

The Fingers on the Trigger

Trust those who seek the truth but doubt those who say they have found it.

—ANDRÉ GIDE, NOBEL LAUREATE IN LITERATURE

We cannot solve our problems with the same thinking we used when we created them.

—ALBERT EINSTEIN

What is really causing your symptoms?

It usually takes more than one insult to result in a disease. While the connection between cause and effect may appear clear-cut—"I eat gluten and get symptoms"—the link may not be that straightforward. There are many triggers of symptoms that are attributed solely to gluten or grains that come from very different sources. The following chapters explain not only some of the newest research into the reasons for both GI and systemic disorders, but also explore the intriguing and nonintuitive links between what we ingest and experience with our GI and mental health.

Some come from left field, such as a drug for blood pressure that inflames the intestine and mimics celiac disease. Others are found in foods that create similar symptoms—the nongluten proteins in wheat, dietary carbohydrates that create bloating. A few are genetic, and, increasingly, research is examining inflammation itself as a potential source of both gut and brain issues.

Finally there is the "double hit," when one condition triggers another—a diagnosis often missed when the initial condition is supposedly successfully treated before the second one occurs. Links are now being identified between parasitic or bacterial infections that predispose to a compromised gut that then becomes sensitive or intolerant to specific foods; childhood abuse, trauma, and alcohol abuse have been identified as triggers of intestinal diseases later in life.

While we all like clear directions—"make a left, follow this road, and in 500 feet you are at your destination"—symptoms come from signals that loop through a jungle of interconnections within the 30-foot-long GI tract.

The following chapters will give you a scientific guidance system to help navigate the maze and reveal what may be triggering your symptoms.

11

Gluten and Nongluten Grains

*An editor is someone who separates the wheat
from the chaff and then prints the chaff.*
—ADLAI E. STEVENSON

In the past number of years the media has accused gluten of aggravated assault and bodily harm. Yet it is increasingly clear that there are many other proteins in wheat besides gluten that may be causing the same set of symptoms blamed solely on gluten. These nongluten proteins are being studied as an additional toxic component of wheat that may be a distinct culprit in celiac disease and other gluten-related disorders.

Which is to say that beneath the chaff, there is more than gluten in the wheat.

Gluten and Nongluten Proteins

Gluten is a term that is used to describe the 70 different "storage" proteins of wheat. Often referred to as gliadins and glutenins in articles or studies, they are the bulk of the protein content. The many enzymes at work in the digestive tract do not easily digest these complex proteins. In people with celiac disease, the partially digested gliadin fragments cross the mucosal lining of the intestine and provoke an immune response. But *many* people are unable to digest gluten well, and this also triggers a response within the GI tract, causing GI symptoms.

Nongluten proteins make up about 25 percent of the proteins in wheat and are often grouped as albumins or globulins. Several of these non-gluten proteins—notably, amylase trypsin inhibitors—may be additional fingers on the trigger.

Wheat Amylase Trypsin Inhibitors

Amylase trypsin inhibitors (ATIs) are part of a family of nutritional proteins found in wheat and related grains that serve a protective function by inhibiting specific enzymes in bacteria and by increasing the plant's resistance to certain pests and parasites. Recent attempts to breed pest-resistant—and therefore high-yielding—wheat have led to a drastic increase of ATI content.

Nongluten proteins were once considered nontoxic for those with celiac disease, but recent studies disprove that assumption. People with celiac disease make antibodies to some of these proteins, such as ATIs, which have recently been incriminated as possibly contributing to the development of the disease. While ATIs do not explain the upsurge in cases of celiac disease, they may contribute to the development of gluten sensitivity. ATIs may be part of a group of nongluten molecules that drive intestinal inflammation.

This family of molecules has also been identified as allergens. They are responsible for wheat allergy and/or baker's asthma. Researchers have therefore focused on these nongluten proteins as possible mediators not only in celiac disease but other GI and nonintestinal inflammatory conditions.

Importance of ATIs in Celiac Disease

The role of nongluten proteins as a trigger of the immune response in celiac disease is a key question since current tests as well as therapies are directed against gluten. The suggestion that ATIs may be toxic may help to identify new targets for both diagnosis and treatment.

The role and significance of nongluten proteins in the development not only of celiac disease but other inflammatory conditions in the gut and body is an important avenue of current and future research. Research into the main nongluten proteins that may cause an immune response—including serpins, purinins, amylase/protease inhibitors, globulins, and farinins—may eventually target additional dietary troublemakers and treatment options.

Oats

I feel empty if I don't start the day with my bowl of steel-cut oats.

(MIMI, 37)

Oatmeal porridge? Even the thought of eating that mush . . .

(CARL, 43)

A bowl of steaming oatmeal has long been advertised as "the perfect way to start the day." Some would disagree. Because of the health benefits of oats—they contain many vitamins as well as fiber—they are also often made into cookies and added to crisp toppings and meat loaves. As a star player in the high-fiber arsenal, oats are praised for their ability to fight cholesterol, help prevent heart disease, lower blood sugar, and help prevent type 2 diabetes. They are also listed as a robust antioxidant.

Because of these many advantages, oats have been studied and accepted as a well-tolerated alternative to wheat for children and adults with celiac disease.

Oats have found their way to our "fingers on the trigger" list because a new study has found a molecular explanation for why some people with celiac disease and others with gluten sensitivities may not be as tolerant of oats as once believed. The inflammation that results may be the source of GI symptoms that are not initiated by but blamed on gluten.

The protein in oats are avenins, which are not thought to cause a reaction in the majority of people with celiac disease. Celiac disease involves a reaction to glutenins (the protein portion of wheat), *hordeins* (barley), and secalins (rye). But antibodies to avenins have been documented in some people with celiac disease.

One possible reason for this enhanced response to oat protein may be a general elevation of food antibodies in an already inflamed intestine. When the gut is inflamed, the normal protective barrier of the intestine (the *epithelium*) can become damaged, and pathogens can travel through and between it and initiate an antibody response. (See chapter 16, "Intestinal Permeability.")

There are a number of other reasons that oats may cause GI symptoms. While oats are safe for most people with celiac disease and gluten sensitivities, cross-contamination during milling and processing can still occur. It is also important to note that because of oats' high fiber content, some people who add oats to their regular diet encounter bloating, gas, and indigestion. This is generally more a result of the sudden addition of so much fiber and usually gradually disappears when your intestines adjust to the change. This is very common for anyone adding any type of fiber to his or her diet—it must be gradual!

We continue to recommend monitoring and follow-up of people with celiac disease and gluten sensitivities who regularly ingest oats as part of their diet to ensure that there is no sensitivity or antibody reaction to this nongluten grain.

Summary

- Your body can develop an immune response to a number of proteins besides gluten in different grains. This immune response does not necessarily mean that these proteins are toxic.
- If other proteins in wheat are involved in the development of celiac disease, they may play a role in its treatment.
- The antibody response triggered by nongluten grains needs to be investigated further. We do not know if they are innocent bystanders, part of a general immune response in the gut of people with celiac disease, or if they may in fact have potential as biomarkers for other gluten-related disorders.

12

Carbohydrates and FODMAPs

Carbohydrates, from the Latin carbo, which means "yummy,"
and hydrates, which means "cinnamon bun," are not
something I can eliminate or even drastically cut back on.
—CELIA RIVENBARK

Most of the energy we need to move and live is provided by the carbohydrates we eat. They are the most readily digested form of fuel for the
body—for most people. For others, carbohydrates often trigger the most
gastric symptoms.

Taken in excess—mainly in processed and manufactured foods sweetened with them—they also fuel weight gain. In some people certain carbs
also fuel a rapid race to the bathroom to deal with diarrhea and flatulence.
For them, carbohydrates are not just fingers on the trigger but a heavy
foot on the intestinal gas pedal.

What Exactly Are Carbohydrates?

All carbohydrates are sugars (saccharides) found in grains, fibers, fruit,
vegetables, plants, roots, and nuts. Manufacturers also add them in a

condensed form (e.g., dextrose, corn syrups/fructose, malt, glucose) to sweeten processed products from breads to soft drinks, canned goods to yogurts, cereals to soups. Catering to the human cravings for sugar, salt, and fat—necessary for body function and survival—the food industry has added sugars to so many products it is difficult to avoid them in the supermarket.

All carbohydrates are classified according to the complexity of their makeup.

- **Monosaccharides** (*mono,* "one"; *saccharide,* "sugar") are the simplest sugars, such as glucose and fructose. Glucose is found in fruits, corn, corn syrup, honey, and some roots; fructose is found together with glucose in honey and fruit. It is commonly used to sweeten products in the form of high-fructose corn syrup.
- **Disaccharides** are two sugars joined together and usually contain glucose. Sucrose is glucose and fructose; lactose is glucose and galactose. Sucrose is table sugar and found in fruits, vegetables, honey, sugar cane, sugar beets, maple, and corn syrup. Lactose is the main sugar found in milk and can be broken down only by lactase.
- **Polyols** (sorbitol, mannitol, and xylitol) are the alcohol forms of some sugars. They are poorly absorbed, if at all, from the GI tract and inhibit a rapid rise in blood sugar, which is why they are often found in products designed for diabetics. While they are found in fruits and plants, they are also manufactured and usually added to sweeten "sugarless" products. People who chew sugarless gum consume a great deal of polyols. Because they are not fully absorbed by the body, they can be a potent cause of diarrhea and bloating.
- **Oligosaccharides** (*oligo,* "a few") contain several sugars and are the fructans and galactans. They are found in plants including

wheat, some vegetables (e.g., onions and the onion family, garlic and asparagus), and legumes (e.g., beans, lentils).

- **Polysaccharides** (*poly,* "many") are the most complex carbohydrates and are starches, dextrin, glycogen, and cellulose. Starches and dextrin are most easily digested and found in plants. Glycogen is the main storage form of glucose in the body. Cellulose is largely indigestible.

Although it is possible to live on a low-carbohydrate diet, carbohydrates are the main source of energy for the brain and for maintaining function in nerve tissue and metabolizing fat. They are also the major food for the trillions of microbiota living in our gut. In this role, carbs have come under attack as a cause of obesity and implicated in various GI conditions such as irritable bowel syndrome.

While most of the sugars in the diet used to be consumed in the form of fruits, grains, vegetables, and table sugar—cooked into homemade baked goods—we now consume most of our carbohydrates from commercially prepared food to which sweeteners have been added.

The Problem with Carbohydrates

After I've eaten an apple or almost any other fruit, I can take a running start out of my driveway and take off without need of a car.

(HARRIET, 33)

As we saw in chapter 7, most of the food we eat is broken down and absorbed in the small intestine. But some sugars and insoluble fiber do not digest easily and arrive in the large intestine (colon) mostly undigested. The wall-to-wall bacteria lining the colon (see chapter 9, "The Microbiome") dine happily on the undigested fiber and sugars presented to them by our diet. This process is called fermentation and produces a great deal of gas and liquid that builds up in the large intestine. The result can be pain and bloating and changes in gut motility (movement). This in turn causes it to empty too quickly (diarrhea) or too slowly (constipation). Recently, researchers have identified a group of sugars/carbohydrates that appear to underlie many of the common symptoms seen by gastroenterologists. They are identified under a new classification: FODMAPs.

FODMAP is the acronym for:

Fermentable
Oligosaccharides
Disaccharides
Monosaccharides
And
Polyols

The FODMAP diet plan is based on avoiding the particular sugars for those people whose symptoms are triggered by them. It essentially removes the food supply for the bacteria in the colon that are creating the liquid, gas, and bloating. In particular, it is effective for quite a number of people with IBS, though not all experts in the IBS field agree with its curative abilities. The diet is individualized to each patient—some are only intolerant to fructose, others a combination of FODMAPs.

Nevertheless, it can be very restrictive as FODMAPs are the basis of a good deal of our foods. There are a number of breath tests (see chapter 6, "Testing") that can immediately diagnose intolerance to a specific sugar and enable patients to include or exclude them from their diet.

The low-FODMAP diet targets and eliminates specific carbohydrates—and is not intended as a cure but simply to control symptoms.

Wheat is an oligosaccharide (a fructan) and a FODMAP. Since many gluten-free products are also low in FODMAPs, people without celiac disease who go gluten-free are also eliminating many FODMAPs. Researchers have shown that the lowered FODMAP content, not the elimination of wheat per se, may be the reason symptoms resolve. This has raised the interesting question of whether people suffering from what is termed *gluten sensitivity* or *intolerance* actually have problems with the digestion of FODMAPs rather than with gluten.

People with celiac disease can also be intolerant to a number of FODMAPs and may need to eliminate them to fully resolve the symptoms.

> The low-FODMAP diet removes many favorite and commonly consumed foods such as milk, garlic, onions, apples, and wheat and can lead to a reduction in fiber and calcium intake. Working with a knowledgeable dietitian ensures the patient is guided through the diet's many nuances, educated not only on appropriate low-FODMAP foods but encouraged to eat a well-balanced, varied, and nutrient-rich diet. When a patient is willing to embark on an elimination diet, they should be given the best opportunity to succeed with the diet plan. The dietitian plays a key role in successful implementation of the low-FODMAP diet education.
>
> —KATE SCARLATA, R.D., L.D.N.

On a FODMAP program, you may also be eliminating a number of vitamin-, calcium-, and fiber-rich foods from your diet. For this reason the diet is best undertaken under the care of a registered dietitian or knowledgeable nutritionist. We will typically advise a strict low-FODMAP diet for several weeks. If it is going to work, it works quickly. Then foods can be reintroduced, because most patients do not have to avoid all FODMAPs.

A low-FODMAP diet is associated with a reduced abundance of bacteria in the colon, while a higher-FODMAP diet showed evidence of stimulation of the growth of bacterial groups with assumed health benefits. In other words, the low-FODMAP diet alters the diversity and reduces the abundance of the microbiome. The significance and health implications of this finding may lead to caution about reducing FODMAP intake for asymptomatic people or even symptomatic people for an extended period of time. More research is needed on the health benefits/drawbacks of any restrictive diet.

Things You Need to Know—It's Not All about Carbs

Bloating, diarrhea, and constipation are very common and can be caused by a number of things, including bacterial overgrowth, lactose intolerance, fructose intolerance, celiac disease, or IBS. Therapies are specific for each condition, and any one symptom can have an entirely different underlying cause.

13

Drugs

For every action, there is an equal and opposite reaction.
—ISAAC NEWTON

Pharmaceuticals to me are as much part of the problem as part of the solution. There's a whole world of things out there. Hidden danger.

(NED, 52)

Most of us ingest an array of drugs to fight disease, aid digestion, control cholesterol and high blood pressure, replace hormones, dull pain, loosen joints, dry acne, grow hair, and elevate mood—to name just a few. While some drugs, such as laxatives, antidiarrheals, and antacids, are meant to affect the GI tract, others have side effects that can seriously alter GI function and impact the body. These drugs include proton pump inhibitors (PPIs) used to control stomach acid, aspirin and other nonsteroidal anti-inflammatories (NSAIDs), immunosuppressants, Benicar (a commonly prescribed antihypertensive), and antibiotics.

Like a seesaw, drugs intended to treat and cure one condition shift intestinal balances and can initiate another. Sometimes this very side effect can be helpful in treating another condition. For example, cholestyramine, a cholesterol-lowering drug, has a constipating effect and is used to treat diarrhea.

Other side effects are subtle, long-term, and obvious only after years of using the drug.

While the benefits of a pharmaceutical drug usually outweigh its potential side effects, an educated patient can better approach and manage GI reactions and ramifications. All of the drugs in this chapter work on and within the normal workings of the GI tract. Some appear to alter the intestinal microbiome, but the meaning of these alterations is still unclear.

It must be reiterated that many drugs have GI side effects. The following drugs stand out for their ability to alter GI function and trigger problems that are often misdiagnosed.

Proton Pump Inhibitors

Proton pump inhibitors (PPIs) are a class of drug that inhibit the amount of acid that your stomach produces. They are used to treat the symptoms of *gastro-esophageal reflux disease* (GERD) as well as other conditions caused by excess stomach acid, such as erosive esophagitis (damage to the esophagus by stomach acid), and ulcers. While PPIs are a blockbuster market for the pharmaceutical industry, most studies demonstrate that they are often used inappropriately.

Stomach acid and PPIs are both two-edged swords—they are beneficial as well as potentially harmful. On one hand, the microbiota of the stomach—*H. pylori* is the dominant microorganism—are comfortable in and accustomed to their unique acidic environment. But *H. pylori* and an acidic environment can encourage the formation of gastric and peptic ulcers.

While PPIs effectively reduce acid, they do not act on the *H. pylori* that causes many ulcers. This bacteria lives under the thick mucous layer of the stomach and is difficult to eliminate. Treatment usually consists of a multidrug regimen including different antibiotics and antibacterials, as well as a PPI (which is necessary for the antibiotics to work).

The greatest clinical benefit of PPIs is to treat GERD. They are so effective that people with GERD may neglect the lifestyle changes that may be all that is needed to prevent GERD symptoms. (See chapter 8.)

But while PPIs efficiently lower stomach acid, they often disrupt the protective effect of the acid from the bacteria we ingest with our food, and increase the risk of *gastroenteritis,* traveler's diarrhea, and *C. difficile* infection. Available both with and without a prescription, drugs such as Prilosec, Nexium, and Prevacid are overused to treat excess stomach acid and, in the process, suppress its natural antibacterial effect. Once stomach acidity is lowered, the effect reverberates down the digestive tract, changing the balance of bacteria into the small intestine.

We have conducted studies on the effects of PPIs, and several interesting findings have emerged. Most important, we found that exposure to PPIs was strongly associated with a subsequent diagnosis of celiac disease. This was found mainly in younger individuals who were exposed to both PPIs and *H2RAs* (histamine 2 receptor antagonists, a drug that reduces the amount of acid produced in the stomach, using a different mechanism than a PPI). While the mechanism by which acid suppression affects the development of celiac disease is unknown, it raises many intriguing questions about the connection of celiac disease to an altered microbiome.

PPIs are given to help eradicate *H. pylori,* prevent and cure ulcers, and treat GERD. However, the long-term use of PPIs also increases the risk of several systemic and GI conditions, including increased risk of fracture, increased pneumonia, low magnesium levels, vitamin B12 malabsorption, and increased kidney disease.

They are a finger on many triggers.

Drugs That Mimic Celiac Disease

Olmesartan

Recently, a patient came into the Center with diarrhea and dehydration severe enough to cause kidney failure and requiring dialysis. The symptoms mimicked an acute and critical form of celiac disease but were, in fact, caused by Benicar (olmesartan), a drug given to lower blood pressure.

Olmesartan can cause intestinal problems that appear to be celiac disease. It is part of a class of drugs called angiotensin II receptor blockers (ARBs). Angiotensin II is a very potent chemical that causes the muscles that surround blood vessels to contract and the vessels to narrow. When blood vessels narrow, the pressure inside increases, creating high blood pressure. ARBs block angiotensin II, allowing the blood vessel to dilate and reducing the pressure. This is a very popular class of antihypertensive medication.

While the GI effect of Benicar is rare, it is a potentially life-threatening situation that should be investigated in anyone taking the drug. It can cause damage to the villi of the small intestine, diarrhea, malnutrition, dehydration, and weight loss. These celiac-like symptoms usually improve dramatically once the drug is stopped.

Immunosuppressants

Also called antirejection drugs, immunosuppressants reduce the strength of the body's immune system, which results in an increased risk of infection and malignancy. All patients receiving an organ transplant take them so that the body will not attack the new organ as "foreign" and reject it.

They are also used to suppress the immune system in autoimmune diseases such as lupus or rheumatoid arthritis, where the body inappropriately attacks its own tissue, or in severe cases of refractory or unresponsive celiac disease and other inflammatory bowel diseases (e.g., Crohn's, ulcerative colitis) to control the intestinal inflammation. With control, the inflammation is dampened, and the gut's powerful ability to respond to pathogens is also inhibited.

Immunosuppressants are classified into four basic categories that include azathioprine (Imuran), cyclosporine, monoclonal antibodies, and corticosteroids (prednisone). Many transplant patients and those suffering from severe IBD take a combination of them.

Immunosuppressants can stop the crippling effect of many autoimmune diseases but can also cause injury in the upper GI tract.

Nonsteroidal Anti-Inflammatories

Nonsteroidal anti-inflammatories (NSAIDs) are the mainstay of OTC treatment for aches and pains of all kinds. This grouping includes aspirin, ibuprofen (Advil, Motrin, Nuprin), naproxen (Aleve), and ketoprofen (Actron, Orudis). They are also prescribed in stronger form by doctors when needed for more acute pain. Many people take "an aspirin a day" to guard against blood clots. For others with arthritis and sports injuries, NSAIDs are part of their daily regimen.

The most common side effects of NSAIDs are GI problems. Since aspirin is absorbed directly into the bloodstream from the stomach, it does most of its damage there. Serious side effects include bleeding, peptic and esophageal ulcers, or perforation.

Some aspirin tablets are available enteric-coated so that they are carried farther down the GI tract, where they are absorbed and supposedly do less damage. But this can cause changes in intestinal permeability. So, while aspirin saves lives by reducing cardiac events, it can be toxic to the epithelial lining of the gut, causing intestinal ulcers or *strictures*.

Many athletes take NSAIDs to prevent anticipated exercise-induced pain. But these drugs also may have a potentially hazardous effect on the GI mucosa during strenuous physical exercise. A small study recently showed that ibuprofen aggravated exercise-induced small intestinal injury and can cause gut barrier dysfunction in healthy individuals. The study concluded that NSAIDs consumed by athletes are not harmless and their use should be discouraged.

NSAIDs should not be used regularly unless under the guidance of a physician.

Opiates

Opiates (prescription painkillers derived from opium) slow down the motility (movement) of the GI tract. This can cause delays down the entire length of the gut and constipation. It can also result in nausea, a feeling of fullness after even a small meal, and bloating.

Antibiotics

Science never solves a problem without creating 10 more.
—GEORGE BERNARD SHAW

Antibiotics are a class of drugs designed to kill or disarm bacteria. They have played a large role in saving lives and changing the average lifespan of people from 49 years in 1900 to more than 78 years today.

Some antibiotics are created to target specific bacteria; others are "broad spectrum" and destroy a range of bacteria. Although they are often taken inappropriately for viral infections such as colds and flu, they do not kill viruses.

But we have paid a price for their use—and overuse. There is a growing array of "superbugs" that are outsmarting our antibiotics. And of particular importance to what is going on in the gut, they often upset the balance of microbiota in the GI tract by destroying "good" as well as "bad" bacteria. Much research is now being conducted on the short- and long-term effects of antibiotics on both body and brain. And the microscope is on the microbiome.

Antibiotics, Allergies, and Obesity Theories

When my daughter was working in the ER, she got TB (tuberculosis). It took something like 12 weeks rather than the usual six for her sputum to test negative. There were pockets of the TB bacteria hidden in little cavities in her lungs, buried in deep, as I understand it. Her daughter has so many allergies—one pediatrician said when my granddaughter was six months old, "this child is an immunological disaster"—and she thinks they are related to all the antibiotics she took during that time.

(MARY, 67)

The prenatal exchange of antibiotics between mother and child may affect the colonization of bacteria in the newborn's gut. Researchers are examining the potential for an association with obesity (the mechanisms are unclear), allergies, and the early use of antibiotics.

There appears to be more diversity in the microbiome of leaner people. This has led to several hypotheses:

- Bacteria could use up calories.
- Antibiotics may cause obesity since they kill bacteria.
- Bacteria could affect the metabolic processes in the body.
- People with less microbiotic diversity are more likely to have a risk for type 2 diabetes, heart disease, and cancer as well as insulin resistance.

It should be noted that these theories are controversial.

Antibiotics and Animals

It has been shown that—for reasons not fully understood—some antibiotics help cattle grow faster, gain more weight, and get more from the feed they ingest. While the prolonged use of antibiotics in cattle and other "food" animals is under scrutiny for the potential side effects to humans eating these animal products, the alteration of bacteria through the use of antibiotics in these animals and the resulting weight gain give evidence to some mechanism related to an altered microbiome. (See chapter 9, "The Microbiome.")

The use of antibiotics on the farm has resulted in antibiotics in our food supply. While the effects are not known, they may be important. The FDA has been studying this issue, and more regulation and research is required to address this potential public health problem.

> My uncle died of a kidney infection in 1928 at the age of 30. If he had
> been born 10 or 15 years later, after penicillin was discovered and in
> use, he would have lived to raise his infant son.
>
> (ROBERT, 75)

It must not be forgotten that antibiotics save lives. They fight lethal infections and keep serious infections from becoming lethal. They are first-line therapy for many deadly infections that are now curable. But they are also misused—when prescribed for minor colds, sore throats, coughs, and infections that turn out to be viral. Patients often take part of a prescription and stop when they "feel better," leaving bacteria behind that becomes resistant to that antibiotic. Or, alternatively, they are taken for too long.

Unexpected Side Effects

> A friend of mine was getting extremely tired. It turned out that the
> pharmacist had filled his prescription for his cholesterol-lowering
> drugs with Valium, which he was taking every day. They were both
> blue pills!
>
> (PAUL, 66)

Some people have individual sensitivities to drugs that can cause a so-called side effect to take center stage. Unfortunately, prescriptions can also be misfilled with a similar-looking pill. Prescription refills should be examined closely to ensure that you are taking the right medicine.

Summary

- Drugs are a major cause of GI symptoms—because of their actions as well as your reactions to them.
- The side effects of many drugs are focused on their first point of contact in the body: the GI tract. The effects then ripple through other parts of the body.
- Older adults who take multiple pill regimens need to be particularly diligent of side effects—many of the pills interact with others.
- When we talk about the mouth, gut, and brain, this includes *everything* we ingest. When asked by a doctor, "What medications or drugs are you taking?" remember to include OTC products even if they are labeled "natural."
- Drugs are self- and doctor prescribed. They cure symptoms and diseases but can often cause others. Before you blame the food you are eating for your symptoms, examine the drugs you ingest.

For every action, there is a reaction.

14

The Double Hit Theory

The game is played away from the ball.

—ANONYMOUS

Diseases are caused by many interacting factors—more is usually involved than exposure to a virus, germ, or food. For example, when someone sneezes in a crowded room, some people will catch that person's cold; others will not. And while most people eat gluten, very few develop celiac disease. Even for people who are sensitive to the grain, gluten alone may be harmless until the body experiences a "double hit," causing a more active reaction to this protein.

The double hit theory explores the relationship between specific infections, illnesses, and conditions that are not caused by gluten yet open the door to a second "hit" or "insult" that creates celiac disease, gluten intolerance, or even diseases of the brain.*

---

* It is a cousin of the "two-hit" hypothesis of Alfred Knudson, which explained the relationship between the hereditary and nonhereditary, or sporadic, forms of one type of cancer.

Lighting the Fuse in the Gut

There are a number of GI conditions that occur after a double hit.

Traveler's Diarrhea

When I was living in South Africa I got giardia. And basically it went undiagnosed. They couldn't figure out what was going on. And they kept giving me antibiotics for treatment. I was terribly nauseated, had skin rashes, bouts of diarrhea. After that I was sick all the time.

Back home, I went to see gastroenterologists, who told me that I had gastritis and my gut was irritated—but that there was nothing really wrong with me. The gastroenterologist actually said to my mom after the appointment that he thought the symptoms were in my head. My mom told him that she had seen how sick I was, and it did not seem credible to her that a healthy 21-year-old wanted to be sick all the time.

It was only when I finally went to see another doctor, who looked at all of my symptoms together—including the rashes, allergies, etc.—that I was diagnosed with a significant parasitic infection and candida.

The healing process from that took a while. (I was dewormed, took probiotics, put on a restrictive diet that included taking me off gluten.) And I started feeling a lot better. Now? Sometimes I still get stomachaches. My tolerance for not feeling great is pretty good. Your baseline is different when you've been so sick.

(JUNE, 32)

Traveler's diarrhea or "turista" is a common complaint of people who leave home and develop gastroenteritis during their trip. For others, parasitic friends also return home with them, requiring numerous courses of drug therapy to erase.

This is a common story after travel to an exotic locale. Caused by different organisms, these GI infections upset normal GI function, possibly disrupt the microbiome, often require rounds of antibiotics or antiparasitics that can in themselves create symptoms, and may set off a chain reaction that results in another GI condition. For those people whose symptoms persist, some will then develop IBD, celiac disease, IBS, or food sensitivities.

But viruses, bacteria, and parasites also attack at home with similar results.

Fooling the Immune System—Gluten and Rotavirus

According to the CDC, rotavirus is the most common cause of childhood diarrhea throughout the world. It produces prolonged diarrhea and is common in preschool children. The CDC studies note that almost every child in the U.S. has had at least one rotavirus infection by the age of 3. The virus attacks the lining of the small intestine, causing inflammation and loss of fluids and *electrolytes*. Once exposed to rotavirus, the immune system "remembers" it.

Evidence that it is a risk factor for celiac disease comes from studies showing that children with celiac disease have a greater number of rotavirus antibodies than those without it. While the mechanisms behind this are not fully understood, one theory is that rotavirus sets up perfect conditions for a double hit because it cross-reacts with gluten through something called "molecular mimicry." Another theory is that gluten disrupts the mucosal barrier, allowing gluten to be recognized as foreign.

Gluten is similar in structure to other proteins in our body as well as some viruses, namely rotavirus. Therefore, when susceptible individuals eat gluten after having the viral infection, the body's immune system attacks the gluten molecule, thinking it is being besieged by rotavirus again. In other words, part of a molecule of one protein resembles a part of a molecule of a totally different protein. The initial infection primes the immune system's "memory" to react—a double hit that creates a sensitivity to gluten.

Lighting the Fuse in the Brain

Toxoplasmosis and Gluten Antibodies

An exposure to *toxoplasmosis*—a parasitic disease that is found in more than 60 million people in the U.S. but usually kept in check by a healthy immune system—may be connected to an immune response to gluten in sensitive people that occurs well after the initial infection.[*]

Toxoplasmosis is the world's most common parasite. Most people with a healthy immune system never develop symptoms—or will have mild, flu-like ones—but it can lead to serious complications in infants born to infected mothers or people with a weakened immune system.

Research has also indicated a direct relationship between infection with this parasite and the development of schizophrenia in people who develop antibodies to gluten. For these people, this immune reaction is recognized as part of the pathology for psychiatric disorders such as schizophrenia, bipolar disorder, and perhaps autism.

This would support a gastrointestinal basis through which a double hit—toxoplasmosis and sensitivity to dietary gluten—might activate certain brain disorders. It is still unclear whether gliadin antibodies are helping initiate the disease, are a product of it, or are markers for other processes contributing to or causing the problems. (For more, see chapter 27, "Schizophrenia.")

Alcohol Ataxia

Similarly, studies have shown that prolonged and excessive alcohol intake can trigger ataxias in the brain and antigliadin antibodies—although it is

---

[*] Centers for Disease Control.

unclear if this is the only factor responsible for the "insult" to the cerebellum, the part of the brain affected.

Ataxia (from the Greek a, "without" and taxis, "order") creates problems with balance, movement, and coordination. It can affect limbs, body, speech, and eye movements. There are many causes and manifestations of the condition, and the association with gluten in combination with alcohol, is an intriguing part of the "double hit."

Alcohol is a common cause of ataxia. A recent study examined patients with alcohol-related cerebellar ataxia to determine whether alcohol also created sensitivity to gluten in susceptible people. Researchers found that antigliadin antibodies were significantly higher in these patients and that the genes associated with celiac disease (HLA-DQ2/-DQ8) were more than double that of the healthy population. They concluded that alcohol-related cerebellar degeneration might, in genetically susceptible individuals, induce sensitization to gluten. This may result from a primary cerebellar insult, but a more systemic effect is also possible. The sensitization may be initiated by the insult to the brain, or other systemic effects. And the duration and amount of alcohol may not be the only factors responsible for the insult to the brain. (For more, see the discussion on gluten ataxia in chapter 22, "Neuropathy.")

Abuse, Trauma, and GI Illness

A history of abuse and trauma has multiple effects on gastrointestinal symptoms and disorders. Dr. Douglas Drossman, an expert who has studied these conditions for the past few decades, noted, "the prevalence of abuse history is greater among those who have more severe symptoms. The pathophysiological features [functional changes associated with or resulting from disease or injury] that explain this association relate to stress-mediated brain-gut dysfunction."

The mechanisms behind this double hit appear to be stress-initiated changes in immune function in the gut due to an impaired ability of the central nervous system to suppress certain stimuli and signals. Insult leads to injury that cascades into ongoing GI disorders. Or the stress may alter nerve cell connections in the brain that lead to GI-related symptoms or the patient's perception of them.

While victims of abuse and those of trauma (including war veterans) are usually seen in a psychiatric context, Drossman explains that it is important that "gastroenterologists and other health care providers . . . understand when to inquire about an abuse history and what to do with that information."

Abuse history is common in GI practice and more prevalent in patients with more severe symptoms. We have similarly shown that people with persistent symptoms after the diagnosis of celiac disease have an increased history of abuse and other psychological factors.

Effects of War Trauma on IBS Development

The federal government commissioned a report by the Institute of Medicine (now known as the National Academy of Medicine) on the impact that deployment in a war zone could have on the mental and physical health of war veterans who served in the Gulf War. The review found sufficient evidence for an association with several specific psychiatric disorders (including PTSD and generalized anxiety disorder), substance abuse, and functional GI disorders such as IBS and functional dyspepsia.

Since more than 50 percent of deployed soldiers in the study acquired acute gastroenteritis, the review concluded that "deployed vets experiencing war trauma who are also exposed to gastroenteritis are at greater risk to later develop IBS."

While knowledge is growing about the role of abuse and trauma in gastrointestinal illness, the reasons for this association are not known. But stress-related brain-gut mechanisms are beginning to be clarified. This is a double hit that highlights the many complex aspects of the brain-gut axis.

Pediatric Autoimmune Neuropsychiatric Disorders Associated with Streptococcal Infections

The acronym PANDAS describes a subset of children with obsessive compulsive disorder (OCD) and/or tic disorders whose symptoms appear to be related to a streptococcus infection. It is an evolving and controversial concept originated in the late 1990s. The proposed mechanism behind this double hit states that the body produces antibodies that attack the streptococcal infection, which cross-react with proteins in the brain that mimic the streptococcal proteins. Repeated strep infections continuously damage the brain, resulting in a chronic psychiatric disorder.

Some researchers feel that the available evidence does not convincingly support the relationship between streptococcal infections and chronic tic disorders. And the autoimmune origin of PANDAS is still being evaluated. A recent study of a group of children and adolescents with PANDAS that looked for other autoimmune conditions—including thyroid function abnormalities and celiac disease antibodies—did not find any statistical difference with a healthy control population.

At this point, we will cautiously note the potential for streptococcal infections to trigger a double hit on the body, initiating a reaction in/on the brain. But PANDAS does not involve gluten, nor will removing gluten from the diet effect any behavioral change.

The Hormone Hit: Pregnancy

Pregnancy is a time of tremendous hormone variation and is also a stress on the digestive system. In order to feed the developing fetus, the mother's blood sugar levels are higher than normal. Usually, the body makes more insulin to metabolize the increased glucose in the bloodstream, but if it cannot, blood sugar levels rise, and this can result in gestational diabetes. Women with gestational diabetes are at a greatly increased risk of developing type 2 diabetes.

Pregnancy is often the tipping point for a diagnosis of celiac disease. It may or may not be the double hit that stimulates a more active form of the disease.

Food for Thought

Developing an immune response to gluten after a history of toxoplasmosis, alcohol abuse, trauma, and certain infections may be the tip of the double hit iceberg. These various conditions cause a level of gastrointestinal or systemic damage or dysfunction that can compromise and weaken it. Then an additional insult triggers another condition in the gut-brain axis.

Is the double hit involved in the increased incidence of celiac disease and gluten sensitivities? The amount of alcohol consumption, prevalence of toxoplasmosis, and/or intestinal infections has not necessarily increased in the past few decades, but perhaps the use of antibiotics, antifungals, and other drug therapies to treat these various conditions has. And they may be agents of change that open the door to further insult. There may be other environmental "hits" that we have not identified.

The connections between what goes through our digestive tract— food, pathogens, alcohol, drugs—and its effect on our body and brain often play out in more than one act(ion).

What is the take-away lesson? Symptoms and disorders often appear in one place but originate someplace else.

The champion hockey player Wayne Gretzky was once asked why he was so successful. He replied, "I skate to where the puck is going to be, not where it has been."

15

Inflammation

Heat not a furnace for your foe so hot that it do singe yourself.
—WILLIAM SHAKESPEARE

I often feel as if my belly is on fire.

(SUSAN, 25)

Inflammation defends and destroys.

The gut exists in a constant state of low-grade, controlled inflammation. This is provided by the very active immune system found within the internal lining of the small intestine, which samples and monitors everything going through. All of the bacteria, viruses, fungi, pathogens, foods, and other substances we ingest are usually controlled this way. But the internal furnace that protects us from our foes often singes its host.

When things go wrong in the gut, the result is impaired GI function and disease. But you also have inflammation that can affect a specific area of the gut or travel throughout the body. This can contribute to abnormal function in other organs, migraines, peripheral neuropathies, and fatigue. The impact of this fire is being actively studied as a potential trigger for many different conditions that affect the brain as well as the gut and body.

What Is Inflammation?

Inflammation is many different things.

Viewed under a microscope, it is an explosion of cells that should not be there. While it can be seen this way, it appears as symptoms that we feel, such as fever, coughs, and chills due to infection, or swollen joints in conditions such as arthritis or fatigue.

It is possible to assess inflammation in the body through changes in the blood that can be measured, most commonly in an elevated white cell count. There are other commonly used inflammatory markers, such as *C-reactive protein* and *erythrocyte sedimentation rate*. But other cellular markers that are released during inflammation and permeate organs—e.g., *cytokines*—are not usually tested for or seen. This is the inflammation that signals the brain to induce a sickness response that includes increased pain and a negative affect (facial and body expression). It is one reason we crawl into bed with a bad flu. The brain and body are working together to heal themselves through rest and sleep.

What Causes the Transition from Low to High Heat?

Inflammation is a final product that can be triggered by many factors and conditions:

- Drugs—aspirin or NSAIDs that break down the intestinal barrier and result in ulceration and inflammation (ironically, these drugs are also used to lower fevers and reduce inflammation in conditions like arthritis)
- Infections
- Autoimmune conditions
- Immune dysregulation—an aberrant response to bacteria

- Toxins (ingesting a corrosive such as lye or drugs in excess such as Tylenol)
- Allergies

In turn, inflammation may contribute to functional issues affecting the hormonal, nervous, or immune systems.

Inflammation in the Gut

A chronic state of inflammation is necessary for the immune system to police the huge surface area of the gut. This is a challenge not only in terms of its vast microscopic area but because this 30-foot-long pipe is open to the world on both ends. Foreign substances are constantly washing through it.

Everything is held in check by cells of the immune system. The microbiome may also be part of the overall protective apparatus. We evolved with these organisms, and they provide a chronic stimulation for the immune system that is protective.

The immune system functions through a complex interaction of innate (born with) and adaptive mechanisms. These two branches of the system "know" to attack certain pathogens, "learn" to attack others—and "mislearn" in autoimmune diseases, where they inappropriately attack the body itself. In other words, they "recognize" the self as something foreign.

The Key Players

Many cells play a role in balancing the inflammatory response of the immune system in the gut and regulating the "temperature" of the GI burner. Of special importance in this very complex system—which is only outlined here—are cytokines, T-cells, and *dendritic cells.* These cells are cited in most articles about celiac disease and autoimmune disorders and offer a fascinating look at how the body "cross talks."

Cytokines are molecular messengers that respond to infection and trigger inflammation. They are chemical "switches" that turn different immune cells on and off. There are a variety of cytokines, such as interleukins, interferons, and growth factors. An explosion of cytokines can be destructive—they are instrumental in starting the cascade of cells that turn inflammatory heat to "high" and cause damage to intestinal villi as well as in different parts of the body. Drugs that block cytokines—cytokine antagonists, like infliximab—are used to treat several chronic inflammatory diseases.

T-cells are a type of white blood cell that circulates around our body, scanning for infections and abnormalities. There are "killer" T-cells and "helper" T-cells. The first type hunts down and destroys cells that have been invaded by "foreign" material such as viruses, bacteria, or cancer. The second type helps to orchestrate both innate and adaptive immunity. They are capable of "remembering" any germ once they encounter it, and they will destroy them if they encounter them again.

Sometimes T-cell responses are inappropriate—they "recognize" cells of the body (self) as foreign and destroy them. This leads to many autoimmune diseases, including celiac disease, type 1 diabetes, multiple sclerosis, and rheumatoid arthritis. They are also responsible for the rejection of a transplanted organ—"recognizing" it as foreign. A lack of T-cells—as seen in HIV/AIDS—can be fatal, as the body is unable to defend itself against infection.

Special dendritic cells in the lining of the mucosa also monitor the contents of the intestine, both to suppress inflammatory reactions against food and to protect against invading pathogens. These messenger cells monitor the "talk" between our innate and adaptive immune system and play a role in allergic food reactions and autoimmune disease.

The development of the microbiome in early childhood may also drive the development of our intestinal immune function and allow us to tolerate the foreign proteins in foods and organisms. The potential mechanisms behind the cross talk between the microbiome, the intestine, and the immune system is under intense study.

Essentially, the digestive tract and its contents engage in a constant immune cross-talk with cells that maintain a protective inflammation. When we ingest something that is perceived as a threat, these cells turn up the heat.

Systemic Inflammation—Gut to Brain?

There is increasing interest in how—and whether—inflammation alters behavior and thought. The fatigue, pain, and withdrawal experienced during acute illness and infection makes evolutionary sense; they enable the body to fight the infection, heal wounds, and conserve energy. It is believed these reactions are a result of inflammation-generated signals to the brain.

However, if these states are prolonged, pain, fatigue, and withdrawal become depression. In conditions such as IBS, chronic inflammation appears to cause the transition from one set of symptoms into depression and chronic pain, but the mechanisms behind this are unclear.

Inflammation is also being actively studied in different neurological conditions such as autism. (See chapter 26.) Because brain tissue cannot be biopsied, researchers examine cerebrospinal fluid and use imaging tests such as PET scans to measure inflammatory markers in this arena.

There is also intriguing work on mice injected with human DNA that shows serotonin may be a possible mediator of inflammation in the brain. This opens the potential for serotonin drugs to help tame GI conditions. (See chapter 10, "The 'Second Brain' in the Gut.")

In disorders such as schizophrenia and autism spectrum disorder

(ASD), systemic inflammation may also include the gut. In this scenario, systemic inflammation could lead to an abnormal immune response to different foods and, in turn, to an increased antibody response to gluten. It may include a breakdown of the intestinal barrier.

Some of the antigliadin antibodies formed in the gut in celiac disease are also found in conditions such as schizophrenia and ASD. These antibodies are not the precise ones found in celiac disease but are nonspecific antigliadin antibodies. It is unclear which is the horse and which is the cart—do the antibodies develop because of a primary gut problem and contribute to the brain problem? Or is the arrow going in the other direction, i.e., altered brain signals affect gut function?

Anti-Inflammation Diets

It is very exciting to think that you can alter inflammation by changing what you eat. Celiac disease is an amazing example of this—withdraw gluten from the diet and you can reverse a devastating autoimmune disease. However, there is little scientific evidence that changing one's diet can similarly affect other diseases.

But since the microbiome is instrumental in controlling inflammation in the gut, some of the so-called anti-inflammation diets may be altering the microbiome—which is what is actually affecting inflammation. While changing the diet can affect the composition of the microbiome—conceivably making it more or less healthy—this has not been translated into any scientifically proven therapeutic diets as yet.

One important exception may be the effect of extreme changes in diet on the inflammation in some patients with IBD. There is evidence from the 1970s that an elemental diet, devoid of fiber and whole food groups and consisting of predigested food components, may control inflammation in some patients. However, current versions of anti-inflammatory diets are little more than "healthy" diets rich in fiber, minerals, and vitamins.

Summary

We understand a great deal about the gut when there is destructive inflammation in conditions such as celiac disease and IBD. Here we can measure and identify inflammation. There are many unknowns regarding systemic inflammation involving the brain.

More research is needed! Anti-inflammatory diets, supplements, and claims are running way ahead of the science.

16

Intestinal Permeability— "Leaky Gut"

Science is the father of knowledge, but opinion breeds ignorance.
—HIPPOCRATES

The so-called leaky gut has gotten a lot of press recently as the trigger for numerous diseases—as well as a potential target for therapies to treat them. It is a term that has been popularized in the alternative medicine literature.

What exactly is leaky gut? Despite popular articles on the subject, there is very little agreement—or good scientific research—about the subject.

Before we can treat it, we need to understand what causes it, what it may trigger, what this really means for our intestinal health, and, what, if any, effect diet has on it.

First, it is important to understand a few terms.

Intestinal Barrier vs. Intestinal Permeability

The intestinal barrier is the huge mucosal surface of the GI tract that protects the body from the billions of bacteria, microorganisms, toxins, and food components that wash through it daily. It functions as a barrier between the external environment and the closely regulated internal environment of the body and is crucial to our health. Conversely, this barrier must open and absorb essential fluids and nutrients to feed the body.

These opposing goals are achieved by a normal functional state described as intestinal permeability (IP). It is the gatekeeper of the intestinal tract.

This permeability allows the body to "sample" intestinal proteins and present them to the immune system, and allows small molecules to pass through the lining of the intestine. Its mechanism is complex, but it is essentially composed of epithelial cells held together by "tight junctions." Layers of water, mucous, and bacteria (microbiota) are additional barriers protecting the epithelial cells. Many factors can alter intestinal permeability, including infection, bacteria, drugs, alteration in the immune system, and stress.

When IP is altered, the result is often referred to as a "leaky gut." **But IP is a constantly changing and normal physical phenomenon.** Many circumstances and conditions cause the tight junctions that line the GI tract to become slightly porous. It occurs in healthy people—during strenuous exercise, stress, and/or the ingestion of medications, alcohol, aspirin or other NSAIDs—as well as in anyone with intestinal disease.

However, there are various degrees of IP, and we know that it is increased in almost any GI disorder and may contribute to other disease states. In fact, IP is often increased in relatives of people with GI disorders who don't have any manifestation of disease—indicating a possible genetic component.

Tests for Intestinal Permeability

There are various tests to measure IP, the most common being the measurement of two nondigestible sugar molecules—lactulose and mannitol. Mannitol is a small sugar molecule and is absorbed easily through the intestinal barrier. Lactulose is larger and more complex and gets taken up only partially—unless the barrier is more permeable.

The degree of IP or malabsorption is reflected in the levels of the two sugars recovered in a urine sample collected over the following hours. Because IP is so naturally variable and affected by multiple physiological causes—alcohol, pregnancy, exercise, drugs—the test must be done in a highly controlled setting. There is controversy about the timing as well as the reliability of these collections.

Altered Intestinal Permeability

As we noted, a number of factors can compromise the integrity of the intestinal barrier—the lining of the GI tract. This includes:

- Intestinal infection and inflammation
- Allergenic foods
- Toxic chemicals
- Drugs
- Lifestyle factors (intense exercise, trauma, stress)
- NSAIDs, including aspirin

Disruption of the intestinal barrier also disrupts—and is disrupted by—the microbiota living throughout the GI tract. When the intestinal barrier is inappropriately breached, it allows substances into the body that it cannot absorb and/or neutralize. The resulting inflammatory reaction causes a cascade of problems that may result in diseases, including inflammatory bowel diseases and celiac disease. Recently, obesity, fatty liver, and metabolic diseases have also been implicated.

Inflammation and Intestinal Permeability

More important, the pathways for unwanted substances into the body are both *through* and *between* the epithelial cell barrier. This is an important point in understanding the so-called leaky gut. The intestinal barrier absorbs nutrients and fluids *through* the cells of the epithelium (see chapter 7, "The

Normal Gut and Digestion"). But proteins can move *through* an inflamed cell as well as *between* the tight junctions opened by inflammation.

In order to treat celiac disease, it is necessary to stop all the gluten from crossing the intestinal barrier. This affects the celiac disease treatments designed to "close the tight junctions" and stop gluten from entering the body. These treatments do not address the gluten entering through the epithelial cells. (See chapter 30, "Nondietary Therapies.")

The Microbiome and Intestinal Permeability

The microbiome is involved in the development and maintenance of the intestinal immune system. Several diseases have been linked to changes in the populations of microbiota that, in turn, alter barrier function.

For example, it is thought that a high-fat diet causes alterations in gut microbiota and increased gut permeability. This may allow the transfer of bacterial products from the GI tract into the body and cause inflammatory reactions that trigger metabolic diseases such as insulin resistance, type 2 diabetes, and cardiovascular diseases. Since the liver is the first site where toxins get through the GI tract, an altered IP may contribute to a fatty liver. It is thought that nonalcoholic fatty liver disease may be a manifestation of altered IP.

Therefore it is tempting to speculate that modifying the intestinal microbiota and the cellular "gates" of the GI tract with drugs, food components, or probiotic bacteria might offer approaches for future therapy of intestinal barrier-related diseases. But the science has not as yet justified the hypothesis.

Autism and IP

A study was recently conducted to determine the occurrence of damage to the gut mucosa in a small group of autistic children with no known intestinal disorders. Using the lactulose/mannitol recovery tests, 43 percent of them showed altered intestinal permeability (versus none of the controls). The researchers speculated that altered IP could represent "a possible mechanism for the increased passage through the gut mucosa of peptides derived from foods, with subsequent behavioral abnormalities." Because of the difficulty in assessing "normal" intestinal permeability as well as the meaning of an altered one, these types of studies require much more extensive research to draw any conclusions about the effect of altered IP on the development of autism.

Summary

- *Leaky gut* is not a scientific term. It is a popularized and somewhat inaccurate name for a normal physiological function—namely, changes in intestinal permeability, which is a feature of intestinal barrier function.
- The realization that the barrier is so important raises the questions of what can disrupt it and how we can improve gut barrier functions—and what role altering gut microbiota may play.
- Gluten is the known dietary cause for increased IP in people with celiac disease and some with diarrhea-prominent IBS, but not in any other condition.
- There are currently no drugs, probiotics, or diet that have been scientifically proven to improve a so-called leaky gut or to treat it. One drug, larazotide, does appear to tighten the intercellular junctions. Its role in various disease states is being studied.
- This area may be a valuable new target for disease prevention and therapy. We need good scientific research, not pseudoscience hypotheses, to explain potentially important concepts like IP.

PART IV

Putting Order in the Disorders

Most of the advice that I've gotten from doctors is: "Whatever works for you, even if it doesn't work." Sort of "just deal with it." One said: "Well, do the best you can. If it's really bad I'll give you an antibiotic." So I tried a gluten-free diet, and that seems to help. Most of the time.

(ELLIE, 28)

As long as your blood tests are good—that's it. As far as he [the doctor] was concerned I wasn't sick. How I felt? Must be nerves . . .

(LYNN, 48)

*A decade ago celiac disease was considered extremely rare outside Europe and, therefore, was almost completely ignored by health care professionals. In only 10 years, key milestones have moved celiac disease from obscurity into the popular spotlight worldwide. Now we are observing another interesting phenomenon that is generating great confusion among health care professionals. **The number of individuals embracing a gluten-free diet (GFD) appears much higher than the projected number of celiac disease patients, fueling a global market of gluten-free products.***

—THE OSLO DEFINITIONS FOR COELIAC
DISEASE AND RELATED TERMS*

---

* A multidisciplinary task force of 16 physicians from seven countries. Published in *Gut* in 2013.

Many people suffering from unexplained symptoms go from doctor to doctor, specialist to nutritionist, Internet blog to magazine article, and back again. When test results fail to uncover a disease or recognizable condition, patients are often sent on their way. And so, they seek out answers on their own. Many are convinced that gluten plays a major role as the solution to or cause of every unexplained symptom from which they suffer.

The actual picture is more complex. Our bodies are filled with feedback loops. To understand one signal or symptom is not enough to grasp either its message or its part in the whole. The conversations between the gut, the brain, and the microbiome are like a party line shared by multiple subscribers. And researchers are listening in with increasing interest.

The following section puts some order in disorders that affect the gut and the gut-brain axis, and explains where the gluten-free diet works and where it does not.

Keep in mind: Your gut has a limited number of ways to tell you it is suffering. Thus, many of the symptoms of one condition resemble others.

17

Celiac Disease

Being on a GF diet is fine now. But it was like drinking out of a fire hose the first few months: completely overwhelming.

(DIANA, 49)

I can talk forever about making sure the restaurant doesn't put croutons on your salad and preparing menus and all that kind of stuff, but that's way down on the list of really major concerns. I don't think that's the hardest part. I'm much more concerned about the risk of autoimmune diseases with celiac. About my daughter getting lupus or scleroderma.

(MARY, 67)

For those with celiac disease, gluten-free exuberance has created a wonderful array of "safe" products that are readily available at grocery stores as well as online and in health food stores. People now have "gluten intolerance," "gluten sensitivity," "gluten allergy," and plain old "glutenitis." These conditions are different from celiac disease, their autoimmune-driven cousin.

What Is Celiac Disease?

Celiac disease is a multisystem autoimmune disorder whose main target of injury is the small intestine. It is caused by an inappropriate immune reaction to gluten, the protein in wheat, rye, and barley, and occurs in 1 to 2 percent of the population worldwide. Most doctors now understand that a patient's migraine headaches, infertility, peripheral neuropathies, and/or blistering skin (among other conditions) may, in fact, be manifestations of this chameleon-like condition.

The digestive tract is a complex and highly efficient system designed to deal with the outside world going through it. To accomplish this, a series of defenses have been built into the GI system. These include:

- an intact lining of cells protecting the border from mouth to anus
- gastric acid that destroys pathogens in the stomach
- the microbiota that "taste" content, determine its status, then sculpt and continually signal the immune system
- immune cells underneath the mucosa that "learn" which parts of what we ingest are friendly and send antibodies to destroy what they perceive as foe
- the enteric nervous system or "second brain" in the gut, which silently regulates and coordinates the stages of digestion to maintain order while engaging in constant cross talk with a network of neurons outside of the tract
- a low level of controlled inflammation that immediately seals off an infected area

When the immune system senses a serious infection or foreign invader, the normally controlled inflammatory process revs up. In people with celiac disease, undigested gluten comes both through and between the mucosal cells lining the tract. It is inappropriately perceived as an invader by the immune cells, who call for the troops (a cascade of white blood cells producing inflammatory cytokines), thereby creating even more inflammation in order to destroy the perceived pathogen. After repeated assaults, the inflammation destroys the surrounding tissue and causes the villi to atrophy and eventually flatten, losing their ability to absorb nutrients. Without the epithelial cell barrier, our immune system begins to make more antibodies to food proteins.

Essentially, the firemen put out the fire, leaving a burned-out building. The small intestine, the main site of nutrient absorption, is damaged and/ or partially destroyed, which can create vitamin and mineral deficiencies and diarrhea. The ongoing inflammation also creates fatigue and many other related symptoms.

The Gut in Flames

The inflammatory response resembles a battlefield with different troops racing to the scene, releasing their chemical weapons and leaving behind collateral damage and debris. If there is not much damage, the body repairs itself. This occurs when we eat spoiled food or get a stomach "bug." The body responds by putting in more inflammation, the problem is dealt with, and the inflammation subsides.

In people with celiac disease, the gliadin molecule gets into the intestinal lining and continually stimulates the inflammatory response. The inflammation will remain high and cause continual damage until the offending toxin is removed.

The intestine will not recover until you interrupt the vicious cycle by taking gluten out of the diet permanently. This allows the inflammation to subside and normal intestinal appearance to return. With the regrowth of the villi, function can return. Until then, the digestive system creates symptoms that reflect the level of damage to the body—it begins to ask or yell for help.

In some cases, the progress of the reaction is gradual; in others it's rapid and dramatic. Symptoms may also wax and wane over a long period of time. While we know the dietary trigger—gluten—we still do not know why only a small percentage of people who are genetically predisposed develop an active form of celiac disease and why it occurs at varying times in their lives.

Symptoms and Complications

There are four major categories of symptoms and complications in celiac disease.

1. **"Classic" celiac disease**

> My dad at the age of 83 lost a lot of weight. He went from 160 pounds to 90-some. The physicians couldn't figure it out. I was on the phone with his doctor and asked if he checked for celiac disease. He said, "Two-year-olds get celiac disease, not someone his age." I asked: "Would you get a biopsy and check for it?" My dad had celiac disease and he recovered, but he never got all his weight back—which was a good thing. He said, "Living with this disease is not so bad. Whenever I get overweight and want to lose a few pounds, I eat a bagel."
>
> (MICHAEL GERSHON, M.D.)

This category describes mild to severe symptoms that predominantly involve the GI tract. The severity of symptoms is related to the amount of intestinal damage and involves GI disturbances including diarrhea, cramps, bloating, lactose intolerance, increased reflux, and dyspepsia.

2. **"Silent" celiac disease**

> I had numerous pregnancy losses, I had elevated liver enzymes, anemia, I had numbness in my hands, and saw numerous doctors who never connected the dots. After I was diagnosed, we had both of my daughters tested. I have a 17- and a 14-year-old. I could have sworn it was the 17-year-old—she had all of the symptoms . . . It was the 14-year-old, who had no symptoms.
>
> The GI who did her procedure was so excited when he met me after the procedure—her intestines were scalloped and so damaged that he hadn't seen anything like that for a while. He couldn't con-

tain his medical excitement. It was sort of like a *Saturday Night Live* sketch.

(DARA, 42)

While GI problems were once considered to be the major manifestation of celiac disease, the more remote effects of malabsorption are now the most common symptoms seen by doctors. These include:

- **Vitamin and mineral deficiencies.** Vitamins and minerals are absorbed in specific sections of the small intestine: vitamin B12 in the ileum; iron and much of our calcium, fat-soluble vitamins, and folic acid in the proximal portion of the small intestine (where celiac disease does much of its damage).
- **Anemia.** The most common cause of anemia in women is menstrual blood loss. In men, it is blood loss through injury or an intestinal problem. People suffering from persistent anemia, especially iron-deficiency anemia, where other underlying medical conditions have been ruled out, should ask their doctors about testing for celiac disease.
- **Fatigue.** Fatigue can be caused by malnutrition and malabsorption of nutrients, inflammation, iron deficiency, vitamin deficiency, other autoimmune disorders, and/or depression. Chronic fatigue should be considered as a symptom of celiac disease. (See chapter 25.)
- **Osteoporosis.** Osteoporosis is a "silent" condition because most people do not know they have thin bones until one of them breaks. Low bone density and osteoporosis are common in patients with celiac disease. Low blood calcium levels are a specific marker for the condition.
- **Neuropathies.** Small-fiber neuropathies and some ataxias are associated with celiac disease. Neuropathies are also associated with inflammation. Many resolve on a gluten-free diet. (See chapter 22.)

3. **Systemic inflammation and autoimmune diseases**

While malabsorption underlies many of the symptoms of celiac disease, the inflammatory process itself is now understood to be a major factor in the development of symptoms. Inflammation, mainly through the increased levels of circulating cytokines, makes people feel unwell.

It is well documented that autoimmune diseases tend to "travel in packs." That is, if you develop one, you are more likely to develop another. It is believed that this is most likely due to a genetic predisposition. Approximately 8 to 10 percent of all type 1 diabetics have celiac disease, and the number may be higher as more patients are diagnosed. Among the celiac disease patients we see, 30 percent have at least one associated autoimmune disorder, compared to 3 percent of the general population.

People with one diagnosed autoimmune disease and unexplained symptoms should explore the possible link with celiac disease.

4. **Malignancies**

People with celiac disease have a twofold greater chance to develop a malignancy than the general population. The malignancies that occur at an increased rate include non-Hodgkin's lymphoma as the main culprit. However, esophageal carcinoma, small intestinal adenocarcinoma, and melanoma are also seen. A gluten-free diet appears to reduce the risk of developing these malignancies to that of the general population after five years of compliance—with the exception of non-Hodgkin's lymphoma, which appears to be associated with a villous atrophy that fails to heal.

Celiac disease was once called "the great pretender." Its many symptoms and manifestations can masquerade as many other illnesses. This is also the reason it is often missed—patients are labeled with another disease that "sticks," and treated for that condition. They continue to eat gluten and remain sick despite treatment.

What Causes Celiac Disease?

We need to rethink the way people get celiac disease. We know that it is a combination of gluten, genes, and environmental factors—but isolating the trigger remains elusive. While we have identified a number of environmental factors that appear to activate or trigger an active form of the condition, no one factor is present in all cases. This is a puzzle that still has many missing pieces.

While the response to gluten in people with celiac disease—and its manifestations and consequences—have been extensively documented in our book *Celiac Disease: A Hidden Epidemic*, the newest areas of scientific study are focused on the underlying mechanisms initiating and driving the immune reaction.

Gluten

You have to be eating gluten to develop celiac disease. It is the only environmental trigger for an autoimmune disease that has been definitively identified. None of us digest gluten completely since it is a large, complex protein that remains mainly resistant to our normal intestinal enzymes. We know that the gliadin protein—the alcohol-soluble portion of gluten—gets into the lining of the intestine in certain individuals and sets off the inflammatory cascade that causes the disease.

Genes

There is a definite genetic influence that is demonstrated by the prevalence of celiac disease in families and in identical twins, but not all of the genes have been conclusively identified. The two specific genes that have been recognized so far are part of the HLA (human leukocyte antigens) class II DQ genes. The HLA genes are the "sentries" of the immune system. They patrol the immune system and identify "self"— belonging to the body—from "nonself"—a foreign substance. We all have slightly different versions of these proteins inherited from our parents. These are the genes that are used to determine organ transplant suitability.

Ninety-five percent of patients with celiac disease have HLA-DQ2, and most of the remaining 5 percent have HLA-DQ8.* In simple terms, specific genetically driven immune cells with these HLA "sentries" are primed to react to gliadin.

While it is absolutely necessary to have either HLA-DQ2 or -DQ8 or the separate components of these genes, they are not sufficient to *cause* celiac disease. They increase the risk in the general population, but different genes have been identified in other populations. More than 40 other genes are seen more often in celiac disease patients than in unaffected people, but we believe that we have identified only about 50 percent of the genetic influences.

Therefore, in order to get celiac disease, you have to have gliadin, and you have to have HLA-DQ2 or -DQ8. Simple enough, but 30 percent of the general population have HLA-DQ2 or -DQ8 lymphocytes yet only about 1 percent get celiac disease. And since not all identical twins and a large percentage in a given family do not have celiac disease, there are obviously other factors at play. There is increasing interest in *epigenetics*—the modification of genes by other, typically environmental factors that may in turn be inherited. These factors have as yet to be studied in celiac disease. (See chapter 33, "Food for Thought.")

The answer is not just gluten and genes.

---

* These are "nicknames" for HLA-DQ2 (encoded by alleles DQA1*05 and DQB1*02) and -DQ8 (encoded by DQB1*0302 and DQA1*03).

Environmental Factors

There is convincing evidence that celiac disease has increased over the past 50 years—not just the rate of diagnosis that lags behind the actual prevalence of the disorder. But why? The presence of the necessary genetic variants has not changed, nor has the type or amount of wheat that is ingested by most people who eat wheat. Therefore other environmental factors must be contributing to this growing percentage of cases.

Infant Feeding Practices

Up until recently, researchers thought that infant feeding practices affected the onset of the disease. However, it will be hard for anyone to continue to recommend the introduction of gluten—specifically at the age of four to six months—since a recent extensive population study did not find that exposure to gluten at this age decreased the risk of celiac disease. Neither did delaying gluten exposure until a child was 12 months old protect him/her from getting celiac disease. This study was a 10-year, multicountry study conducted in Europe, prompted by the Swedish celiac disease epidemic study of 2001.

The researchers also did not find any evidence that breast-feeding, the duration of breast-feeding, or the introduction of gluten during breast-feeding influenced later development of celiac disease. Although we recognize the overall importance of breast-feeding for child health, breast-feeding does not appear to protect against celiac disease in children. While these European guidelines still appear in the popular press, the recommendation needs to be changed.

Infections

Infections—both in adults and children—may play a role in the development of celiac disease. When the lining of the intestine is disrupted by an infection, some larger molecules such as gliadin can get through the intestinal barrier and set off the immune reaction. Rotavirus infection in childhood and *campylobacter* infection in adulthood (a common food-borne illness from raw or undercooked poultry) both increase the risk of celiac disease. (See chapter 14, "The Double Hit Theory.") Interestingly, infection with *H. pylori* appears to be protective against the disease.

Drugs/Antibiotics/Proton Pump Inhibitors

Drugs and antibiotics can damage the intestinal lining, making it more permeable and more susceptible to food antigens. Just having an altered pH may alter the digestion of gluten. Medications also upset the delicate balance of our microbiome, and that may be a precipitating factor.

Aspirin and Other NSAIDs

Many people are taking enteric-coated aspirin that dissolves in the small intestine instead of the stomach. This transfers the damage from the stomach—where it can cause ulcers and bleeding—to the small intestine. It alters intestinal permeability and may increase the risk of other diseases such as CD. Other NSAIDs, widely available over the counter and used extensively for pain control, also disrupt the intestinal barrier and may play a role in the development of altered intestinal permeability and concurrent disease.

The Microbiome

As we discussed in chapter 9, "The Microbiome," there are many factors that influence the colonization of the microbiota in our gut, including birth mode, antibiotic use, diet, and early environment. Since exposure to microbes "educates" and helps shape the immune system, the initial flora that colonize the GI tract may have important consequences in a child's tolerance to food antigens. While there are no studies that demonstrate a direct relation between a disrupted microbiome and CD, it has been proposed that some microbiota may influence the immune response to gliadin in genetically predisposed individuals. In other words, alterations in the composition of intestinal flora may play a role in the loss of tolerance to gluten. This may be of particular importance during the first few years of life, when the immune system is maturing and being "educated."

Since it has been hypothesized that the intestinal microbiota is somehow involved in celiac disease, probiotics are appearing as an interesting enhancement in the dietetic management of the disease. We do not currently advise them because of the total lack of supporting evidence and regulatory oversight. (See chapter 5, "Supplements and Probiotics.")

Testing Gluten and the Microbiome

We are currently conducting a study to determine the effect of gluten on the microbiota of people with and without celiac disease. Using a gluten challenge, and testing skin and stool microbiota, we hope to have specific answers to its effect. We know that simple dietary modulation may alter the microbiome. What we do not know is whether this is beneficial, neutral, or harmful.

The composition of the microbiome and its role in immunity and celiac disease is an exciting new area of exploration and may be an important piece of the celiac disease puzzle.

An Allergic Component?

Recent studies have shown an increase in eosinophils (white blood cells that control mechanisms associated with allergies) in patients with active celiac disease. They subside on a gluten-free diet, suggesting that there may be an allergic component to the immune response in celiac disease. (See chapter 21, "Eosinophilic Esophagitis.")

Smoking

There are studies that suggest smoking may be protective for celiac disease, and others where this is not confirmed. There are many chemicals in cigarettes besides nicotine, but nicotine patches have been used as "drug" therapy in conditions such as severe ulcerative colitis. While the mechanisms of action are still not completely understood, the therapeutic effect of nicotine appears to dampen inflammation and the immune response. Nevertheless, this does not change the very negative effect of smoking on overall health.

Vital Wheat Gluten

Another factor that has so far received little attention is vital wheat gluten. Processed from wheat flour, this form of gluten is increasingly used in the preparation of baked goods and processed foods. It was investigated in a European multicenter study, and although that study showed negative results, the role of vital gluten needs to be explored further.* (For more, see chapter 31, "Eating Healthy.")

Stress, Life Events, and Trauma

I had a very successful but stressful career. I've always taken things emotionally home with me. I believe there has to be some trigger [for celiac disease]; maybe it's age or something else, but I think that it's stress. I was going through a very stressful period at work, the politics, a boss dying. That's when things really got bad.

(NED, 60)

---

* Of note: The amount of gluten administered to the children in the study was very low (about 2 to 3 percent of the amount of gluten in a slice of bread).

Many patients pinpoint a stressful occurrence as the "triggering" event for their celiac disease diagnosis. A recent study showed that life events may favor the clinical appearance of celiac disease or accelerate its diagnosis.

Stress can be both physical and emotional. While biological stress seems to contribute to the improper functioning of immune cells, the "second brain" in the gut may also play a role in signaling the immune system during emotional stress.

Stress may also affect the protective responses in the gut and create an improper discrimination between pathogens and our microbiota. But to date, only animal models have shown that stress alters the microbiota.

Trauma and pregnancy may also be factors contributing to GI conditions, including celiac disease. (See chapter 14.)

The Mismatch Theory

The mismatch theory lies at the core of evolutionary biology/medicine, a field that applies evolutionary practices to health and illness. It suggests that we are developing illnesses that were previously rare because our bodies possess features preserved by natural selection and designed for survival in a given environment that is unlike the modern environments we have now created and live in. These environmental changes have altered how the body functions.

> *Put simply, mismatches are caused by stimuli*
> *that are too much, too little, or too new.*
> —DANIEL E. LIEBERMAN, *THE STORY OF THE HUMAN BODY*

This theory has been narrowed into a hypothesis that we are eating a food (wheat) that we were not designed or evolved to eat. A number of anthropologists, archaeologists, and molecular biologists have countered this hypothesis based on the so-called Paleo diet:

> *Our bodies have adapted over time to different circumstances,*
> *including to cooking and to modern agriculture, and this process*
> *is always ongoing. There is no pristine virtue in what our*
> *ancestors ate in Palaeolithic times, and in any case our bodies*
> *have already undergone significant changes since that time. Life,*
> *especially human life, is never perfectly matched to one kind*
> *of eating. It is always evolving as the food sources change.*
> —DIMITRA PAPAGIANNI, PH.D., AND MICHAEL MORSE, PH.D.,
> COAUTHORS OF *THE NEANDERTHALS REDISCOVERED*

Ninety-eight percent of the worldwide population that regularly eats glu-ten does not get celiac disease. If you factor in other related gluten sensi-tivities and intolerances, 70 percent of this population has no GI distress from the grain at all.

> *Tomatoes, peppers, squash, potatoes, avocados, pecans, cashews,*
> *and blueberries are all New World crops, and have only been on*
> *the dinner table of African and Eurasian populations for probably*
> *10 generations of their evolutionary history. Europeans have been*
> *eating grain for the last 10,000 years; we've been eating sweet*
> *potatoes for less than 500. Yet the human body has seemingly adapted*
> *perfectly well to yams, let alone pineapple and sunflower seeds.*
> —DR. KARL FENST, BIOARCHAEOLOGIST

Temporary Gluten Autoimmunity—a Confounding Factor

Adding mystery to the puzzle are the children and adults with celiac dis-ease antibodies that go away when they continue on a regular diet. While we feel that this is a rare event, it has been seen in children involved in long-term studies. It is one reason that asymptomatic children tested during a screening should have a second blood test prior to subjecting the child to an endoscopy.

Although this is rarely seen in adults, we did a study on a baker who had positive blood results for celiac disease but a negative biopsy, and whose blood tests normalized on a regular diet after a period of time. It does not appear to occur in patients who have abnormal biopsies.

What does it mean? It means that the switch can go on and then it can go off. But it is very risky to assume that celiac disease has "gone away" since being able to "tolerate" gluten is not a reliable test of whether celiac disease has gone away.

The long-term effects of positive blood tests that switch to negative remain unclear, and these patients should be followed into adulthood. Perhaps we should call these people "potential celiacs."

The danger rests in people who focus on the word *temporary* and go back on a regular diet, only to suffer complications from the continued inflammatory reaction in their GI tract. There are patients in their 50s who were diagnosed with celiac disease as babies, whose parents were told it had gone away, and who ate gluten without symptoms for 40 years—and then developed intestinal cancer.

Management—Diagnosis and Treatment

There have been several advances in the diagnosis of celiac disease in the past few years. Some of the issues of the past, such as variation in lab and pathology interpretation, still lead to incorrect diagnoses.

The panel of tests available for celiac disease includes all of the following. While there are no tests that are 100 percent specific and sensitive for celiac disease, some of the following are extremely accurate.

Diagnostic Tests

1. **IgA tissue transglutaminase (tTG):** tTG is the enzyme that converts gliadin into a more toxic molecule. We consider this one test the "gold standard" blood test. It may be combined with the deamidated gliadin peptide (DGP) to increase the number of diagnoses.

2. **IgA endomysial antibodies (EMA):** This test adds specificity to the diagnosis. (This means that there are no other conditions that can cause a positive result.) It is an expensive test that is read manually by an expert technician. It has been advocated to replace the biopsy in the new European diagnostic pathways for children. (See opposite.)

3. **Total IgA:** This test is not done routinely, as it is unclear whether it is cost-effective. While it is helpful in finding people who are IgA deficient, that is a small group. (**IgG tissue transglutaminase** is used to diagnose celiac disease in IgA-deficient individuals. There is no role when IgA is normal.)

4. **IgA deamidated gliadin peptide (DGP):** The deamidated gliadin peptide test has been developed recently and replaced the antigliadin antibody (AGA) test, which is no longer available. The test looks for specific antibodies that have developed in response to gliadin (the protein portion of gluten). The DGP may not be as valuable as the tissue transglutaminase test, but it is part of the panel that we recommend for celiac disease screening. This test may be positive in some patients with celiac disease who have negative IgA tTG tests.

Biopsy Results

If blood tests are positive, the diagnosis is confirmed with a biopsy. None of the blood tests are either 100 percent sensitive or specific for celiac disease, which is why we still recommend a biopsy as the ultimate gold standard for diagnosis.

Biopsy is pathologist dependent, and not all pathologists are expert at interpreting small intestinal biopsies nor use a standardized terminology for grading the changes in celiac disease. The Marsh score is one such form. If there is a question about the result, the biopsy can always be reviewed by a different pathologist.

False Negatives/False Positives

False negatives: You can have celiac disease and still have negative blood tests, and you can have negative blood tests and develop celiac disease later in life. If you are not eating a lot of gluten, you can have celiac disease with negative antibodies.

A Word on Sensitivity and Specificity

Testing criteria are based on the sensitivity and specificity of the test. These terms are often used in the medical literature, so it is important to understand their meaning.

Specificity: If a test is 100 percent specific, it means there is nothing else, no other medical condition that can cause the positive result.

Sensitivity: If a test is 100 percent sensitive, it means that everyone with the disease has a positive test.

However, no test is 100 percent. Blood tests are designed to have cut-offs that will include most people with the disease. However, they will include some as positive who do not have the disease if they fall in this range, and miss others who do not.

European Pediatric Guidelines

There are pediatric guidelines in Europe that suggest that you can diagnose celiac disease without a biopsy. They are not accepted in the United States. They were created in response to parents reluctant to subject children to a biopsy that is usually conducted under general anesthesia. If used, they require very strict guidelines that need to be adhered to.

The European guidelines require **all** of the following conditions:

The child **must be symptomatic** and then have:

1. A positive tTG more than 10 times the upper level of normal
2. A second blood test for EMA that is positive and that *must* be taken on a separate occasion
3. Presence of genetic markers.

The second blood draw guards against temporary gluten autoimmunity and may account for "false positive" antibody tests. When these criteria are met, a presumptive diagnosis can be made and a gluten-free diet started.

There are pros and cons to these guidelines. On one hand, you diagnose most cases of celiac disease. It eliminates an invasive endoscopy and biopsy, as well as the concern about general anesthesia, which has been suggested as a contributing factor to some cognitive impairment in the very young. However, this has not been conclusively demonstrated. Conversely, the guidelines must be adhered to strictly, and some doctors do not do a separate blood draw, which may not catch children who are asymptomatic. Without an endoscopy, other conditions that occur with celiac disease may be missed. And some children with positive blood tests may not have celiac disease.

We favor being very certain because as the child becomes an adolescent, then an adult, he or she or their adult physician may not believe the diagnosis.

One patient who had been diagnosed with celiac disease as a child by his pediatrician discovered as a young adult that he did not have it. His anger toward his parents when he found out that the childhood diagnosis—done without a biopsy—was not correct remains troubling.

Gene Testing

In any one individual there are multiple factors in addition to genetic makeup that will lead to celiac disease, and they are different for each person. Having the gene(s)—specifically HLA-DQ2 and -DQ8—merely means that you are at risk. However, you must have these specific genes to have celiac disease.

HLAs are human leukocyte antigens, the proteins found on the surface of almost every cell in the body. They are the sentries that patrol the immune system identifying other cells as "self" or "nonself"—a foreign body. These are the genes that must "match" to determine compatibility for an organ transplant.

People should not have a genetic test unless they understand the significance of the test. It is not a determinant of celiac disease and cannot be used to diagnose it. Its value is in a negative result because this excludes the possibility of having the disease. If you have been correctly diagnosed with celiac disease you do not need a gene test.

Approximately 30 percent of people in the U.S. have these HLA-DQ2 and -DQ8 genes, and only 1 percent have celiac disease. It is necessary but not sufficient for development of celiac disease.

Gene testing should be conducted and interpreted by doctors who understand its significance. Home testing, because of the potential for misinterpretation, is not recommended. The presence of these genes is not a reason to commence a gluten-free diet.

The role of genetic testing is to:

- Determine which family members to screen for celiac disease. There is no point in testing family members in an "at risk" family without the genes.
- Diagnose patients in whom antibody and biopsy results appear incongruent.

Point-of-Care/Finger-Prick Testing

Point-of-care testing involves technology that gives an immediate result. These tests can be performed in a doctor's office or purchased commercially without any medical personnel input.

There is a great deal of precedence for point-of-care testing—notably in pregnancy, strep, and HIV kits. Such a test has been developed for celiac disease and currently approved for use in Canada as an OTC product. Because interpretation is particularly important in celiac disease, confirmation with an endoscopy is still necessary. The test is marketed and used in Canada to track a gluten-free diet.

Fecal Testing

Currently, fecal stool tests for celiac/gluten antibodies are neither specific nor sensitive enough to be used as a diagnostic tool. Some labs offer them, but there are *no* rigorous scientific studies proving their validity, efficacy, or usefulness. They have no role in the diagnosis of gluten-related disorders.

Treatment

The current treatment for celiac disease is a lifelong gluten-free diet, though nondietary pharmaceutical treatments are being developed to eliminate the toxic effect of gluten on the intestines of susceptible people. The exact role of these adjunctive therapies remains to be seen, but most will not replace a gluten-free diet. (See chapter 30, "Nondietary Therapies.")

Patients often opt out of further treatment once they are diagnosed and on a gluten-free diet, but the management of celiac disease should not stop at the end of your fork. Celiac disease is a chronic condition like diabetes or high blood pressure and should be monitored with yearly visits to a physician specifically for the celiac disease, to prevent long-term complications.

L-Carnitine

There is a study showing that L-carnitine is effective in the treatment of some types of fatigue found in celiac disease. Supplementation can be very helpful in patients with fatigue and low levels of L-carnitine in their blood. (See chapter 5, "Supplements.")

L-carnitine is an amino acid (a building block for proteins) that is produced by the body and is a natural component of the diet. If tests show that you are deficient in this metabolite and cannot correct this through diet, you should take supplements under a doctor's instruction. It is not a cure-all for the fatigue found in celiac disease.

Summary

- Incidences of celiac disease appears to have increased over the past 50 years. While some risk factors have been pinpointed, others remain to be uncovered.
- Despite intensive research in the past decade, the mechanisms behind celiac disease remain a challenge, and it is still under-diagnosed.
- The variability of age at the onset of symptoms is still puzzling, as well as the variability of the symptoms themselves.
- While many of the environmental factors may be related, they are not necessarily causal. An infection, drug, or life event may uncover the underlying condition rather than trigger it. This is of particular interest as scientists investigate the role of the micro-biome in diseases such as celiac disease. While alterations in the small intestine microbial composition have been associated with

active celiac disease, there have been no studies demonstrating a causative effect to these changes.

- We continue to search for the "switch"—the genetic/epigenetic, environmental, infective, or physiological button—that causes someone to go from tolerating gluten to not tolerating gluten, so that we can prevent it.

We have come a long way, but many intriguing puzzle pieces are still missing.

18

Gluten Sensitivity—the New Kid on the Block

I became gluten-free in 2003 because I was feeling really awful most of the time. I was distended and bloated; my [throat] was always burning. A friend suggested I stop eating bread, and within three days, I noticed a huge difference. I haven't had real bread since then. When I eat it I feel terrible. Instead, I eat a variety of gluten-free grains like rice, corn, and quinoa.

(INGRID, 64)

Nonceliac gluten sensitivity (NCGS) is a new, emerging entity that encompasses a diverse group of conditions that all appear to improve when gluten is removed from the diet. It is unclear how long it has been around, but patients have been aware of it for years. In 2011 a consensus conference established the definition of NCGS within the framework of other gluten-related disorders in the medical community.

It is, without doubt, a popular name in the consumer press. While there are some people with gluten-sensitive symptoms, it is currently a self-diagnosis since **there is no definitive test to confirm its presence.** It is a common diagnosis by nontraditional medical practitioners.

However, the number of patients who have neither celiac disease nor a wheat allergy, but appear to derive benefit from a gluten-free diet, has increased substantially.

What Is NCGS?

NCGS is defined as a reduction in symptoms after eliminating gluten-containing products from the diet and a recurrence of symptoms when gluten is re-introduced in people without celiac disease and a wheat allergy. People with NCGS do not have the small intestinal damage or develop the antibodies (tissue transglutaminase, tTG) found in celiac disease. While it is important that celiac disease is ruled out in these patients, it is worth noting that most people with gluten sensitivity have not been tested for celiac disease or other possible causes of their symptoms.

It is the "youngest" member of the family of gluten-related disorders and is characterized by a great variability in symptoms and clinical history. Most patients report both GI and non-GI symptoms (especially fatigue or "foggy brain") that improve on a gluten-free diet.

The gastrointestinal symptoms are similar to symptoms of irritable bowel syndrome and include bloating, gas, diarrhea, constipation, abdominal pain, and nausea.

The extra-intestinal symptoms include lack of well-being, tiredness, headache, foggy mind, numbness, and joint or muscle pain.

The rapid disappearance of symptoms on a gluten-free diet and their recurrence after gluten reintroduction are also characteristic of the condition.

After a thorough medical evaluation, we find that many PWAGs (people who avoid wheat and gluten) have a variety of other conditions such as lactose or fructose intolerance, bacterial overgrowth, or microscopic colitis and once those are diagnosed and treated they are able to eat gluten again symptom-free. **Thus, a self-diagnosis of NCGS may mask other conditions**. It is also unclear whether another component of wheat is causing symptoms in these people. (See the following section.)

Patients often identify other foods that cause symptoms—50 percent of NCGS/PWAGs seen at the Center are avoiding dairy, soy, or corn as well as wheat.

What Causes NCGS?

Nongluten Components of Wheat?

While NCGS appears to be directly related to an adverse food-related reaction, recent studies suggested that gluten may not be the only trigger, and that different proteins found in wheat (e.g., ATIs) are likely to play a relevant role in this condition.

New studies have shown that a diet low in FODMAPs results in improved symptoms in some patients with self-reported NCGS, supporting the hypothesis of a major role of FODMAPs compared to gluten.

Other possible causes of symptoms in NCGS are wheat amylase trypsin inhibitors (ATIs), other proteins found in wheat and related grains. (See chapter 11, "Gluten and Nongluten Grains.")

Because it is unclear which components of wheat-based products are responsible for an individual's symptoms, it may be premature to assign all of the blame to gluten. This is why we and others prefer to call these individuals PWAGs, as the term better encompasses the possible underlying dietary culprits.

Genes?

Although celiac disease is characterized by a strong genetic association—about 95 percent of patients carry HLA-DQ2, and the remaining 5 percent carry HLA-DQ8—only about 50 percent of patients with NCGS carry HLA-DQ2 and/or HLA-DQ8. Nevertheless, this percentage is slightly higher than the general population (30 percent). This serves to further emphasize the need for patients to be assessed prior to going gluten-free. This is especially important as we learn the pitfalls and hazards of a gluten-free diet. (See chapter 4.)

As the cost of DNA sequencing lowers, it will be interesting to characterize the genetic profile of different subgroups of patients with NCGS.

Management of NCGS

Diagnosis

As noted earlier, there is currently no diagnostic test for NCGS. It is often a diagnosis of exclusion—patients do not have specific celiac disease markers or intestinal damage (villous atrophy), nor do they have high blood levels of IgE indicating a wheat allergy.

An intestinal biopsy sample should always be obtained from patients with suspected NCGS while they are eating gluten to exclude the presence of villous atrophy, the hallmark of CD. About 60 percent of NCGS patients have normal intestinal mucosa.

Some interesting results are starting to appear in regard to the antibodies found in patients with NCGS. Various studies have found IgG anti-gliadin antibodies in a large percentage of patients with NCGS. As explained fully in chapter 6, antigliadin antibodies are targeting gliadin, the protein portion of gluten. While these antibodies are found in celiac disease, these are not the specific IgA antibodies found in celiac disease.

Interestingly, after patients with NCGS started a gluten-free diet, the IgG levels returned to normal in almost all of them. Strict compliance and a good response to a gluten-free diet, with significant improvement in symptoms, were significantly related to the disappearance of IgG antigliadin levels in these patients.

Still, IgG antigliadin cannot be considered a reliable biomarker of NCGS because it is also found in people with many other disorders, including autoimmune diseases, autism spectrum disorder, and ADHD, as well as in healthy subjects. (For more, see part V, "The Brain-Gut-Gluten Connection.") These antibody tests are only available right now in a research setting.

Treatment

It is important to avoid self-diagnosis. If you think you have NCGS you should be tested for celiac disease as well as bacterial overgrowth, microscopic colitis, and other food intolerances and perform a trial of the FODMAP diet before starting—or continuing—a gluten-free diet. A full medical history regarding drugs (both OTC and prescription) should also be taken. NSAIDs and other drugs have been associated with similar symptoms in patients.

A self-diagnosis of NCGS can mask other serious conditions that can affect your long-term health.

Summary

- Patients suffering from NCGS are a diverse group, composed of several subgroups, each characterized by a different clinical history, and, probably, clinical course.
- None of us fully digest gluten the way we digest other proteins such as those in meat, but only 1 percent of people develop an autoimmune response. It is possible that the group with NCGS is a middle group that does not get the full immune response characterized by celiac disease, but develops a greater response than someone with some gas or burps. There may also be a group of NCGS patients who develop villous atrophy in the future.
- A diagnosis of NCGS can only be made by excluding celiac disease and a wheat allergy.
- It is important therefore that we look at ways of better classifying patients with NCGS. An accurate diagnostic test would certainly provide the best way of doing this. Gliadin antibodies and HLA

DQ2/DQ8 genes are more prevalent in NCGS patients than the general population, and it may be that they play a role in delineating NCGS patients in the future, but as yet they cannot be used in diagnosis.

- We need to examine what is triggering symptoms—is it the gliadin proteins, nongliadin gluten parts in grains, gluten contaminants, other wheat constituents such as amylase trypsin inhibitor (ATIs), or only carbohydrates (lactose or fructose) in the diet?
- Future research should aim to identify the biomarkers for a diagnosis of NCGS diagnosis and better define the different NCGS subgroups.

In the past few years, NCGS has become increasingly recognized, and researchers are just beginning to define this entity.

19

Irritable Bowel Syndrome

Let me put it this way: IBS makes me feel as if someone is "fracking" my gut. Massive pressure is injected, enormous amounts of natural gas is forced to the surface, and the effect on the environment is undesirable to lots of people.

(GENE, 55)

Irritable bowel syndrome (IBS) interrupts a life. The symptoms are unpredictable, the pain can be crippling, and patients echo the challenges of airplane travel, family occasions, disrupted meetings, and the psychological burdens they carry.

What Is IBS?

IBS is a functional bowel disorder—which is to say that symptoms are caused by changes in how the gastrointestinal tract works. The GI tract continues to look normal—it appears undamaged—but creates symptoms. It is one of the most common disorders diagnosed by doctors and affects as many as 5 to 20 percent of people worldwide. It occurs more often in women and affects children as well as adults. Symptoms range from diarrhea to constipation—and can yo-yo between both—as well as abdominal discomfort or extreme pain, bloating, and gas. While the symptoms are common, it is unclear why they have such an intense impact on some people and not others.

Some people complain of daily distress while others have intermittent symptoms that may not occur for weeks or months. A decreased quality of life is well documented. While some studies show that only a minority of people who suffer seek out medical care, other patients go to numerous doctors and undergo endoscopies, colonoscopies, X-rays, scans, blood tests, and biopsies—the results of most of which are normal, confounding both patient and physician.

IBS is usually classified into four categories that also determine the type of treatment used for symptoms. These are:

1. **IBS with constipation (IBS-C)**—mainly hard or lumpy stool
2. **IBS with diarrhea (IBS-D)**—mainly loose or watery stools
3. **Mixed IBS (IBS-M)**—a combination of hard and watery stools
4. **Unsubtyped IBS (IBS-U)**—insufficient criteria to meet any of the other categories

It is not uncommon for patients to switch subtypes over time. There are also conditions that resemble IBS. These include functional constipation, diarrhea, and bloating syndromes.

How Is It Diagnosed?

Irritable bowel syndrome is diagnosed through a combination of the Rome III criteria, a physical exam, and tests to diagnose or rule out other conditions with similar symptoms. These include IBD (e.g., colitis, Crohn's disease), celiac disease, ulcers, SIBO, food allergies and intolerances, pancreatic insufficiency, microscopic colitis, or a chronic GI infection or parasite. It is essentially a diagnosis of exclusion.

Nothing in my life is predictable—I never know if I can get through
a concert or a phone call without rushing to the bathroom.

(JANET, 70)

The Rome III Criteria

The Rome III criteria require that patients have had recurrent abdominal
pain or discomfort at least three days per month in the last three months,
associated with two or more of the following:

- Relieved by defecation
- Onset associated with a change in stool frequency
- Onset associated with a change in stool appearance

They must also have symptoms to support the diagnosis, which include:

- Abnormal stool frequency (greater than three bowel movements
  per day or less than three bowel movements per week)
- Abnormal stool form (lump/hard or loose/watery stool)
- Abnormal stool passage (straining, urgency, or feeling of incom-
  plete evacuation)
- Passage of mucus
- Bloating or feeling of abdominal distension

Patients with IBS also report fatigue, a "noisy" abdomen (borborygmi),
and depression. IBS can also occur along with other conditions including
IBD and celiac disease. Symptoms that include fever, weight loss, or blood
in the stool demand a prompt clinical evaluation.

Few clinicians correctly label patients according to the Rome Criteria.
Thirty percent of the patients we have diagnosed with celiac disease had
a previous misdiagnosis of IBS.

There is considerable interest in the development of biomarkers for IBS. Several blood tests are promising, but the biomarkers tested overlap with and are elevated in other conditions, especially celiac disease. Thus, blood tests are not as sensitive for a diagnosis of IBS.

> What's normal for you may not be normal for everyone else. I can't wear certain clothes because my belly blows up when I eat. That's my normal.
>
> (CASSIE, 51)

Unfortunately, patients with IBS usually present with GI complaints for which their doctor can find no organic cause. This has led to diagnoses of psychiatric disorders, hypochondria, and "hysteria." It also forced many patients to ignore symptoms and regard them as a normal part of life. With our growing understanding of the "second brain" in the gut and gut-brain interactions, this perspective has begun to change.

What Causes IBS?

IBS is an extremely prevalent but poorly understood condition—its symptoms distinct, its causes more elusive. They appear to be a complex construction of:

- Genes (people often say that "bad stomachs run in my family")
- Diet and food sensitivity
- The microbiome—a makeup uncharacteristic of gut bacteria from that of healthy individuals
- Infections and/or with antibiotic therapy causing a "double hit"
- An abnormality of bile salt metabolism
- Altered GI motility (how the GI tract deals with and eliminates its contents)
- Brain-gut signaling problems (including a hyperreactivity to stress or psychosocial factors)

Right now, even the puzzle pieces keep changing shape in this complex and challenging condition.

Genes

IBS tends to "run in the family." It is common to hear comments such as "My mother had stomach issues, I've got belly issues, and my daughter pops antacids." While no specific genes have as yet been definitively identified, interesting studies regarding polymorphisms (anomalies) in genes that encode gut serotonin have been implicated.

Studies examining the environment and social learning suggest that the reinforcement of illness behavior in a family can contribute to the heightened awareness of GI symptoms.

Diet and Food Sensitivity

Many patients feel that certain foods trigger their symptoms. In particular, milk and dairy products, spicy or fatty foods, gluten, high-fiber vegetables and grains (cabbage, beans), caffeine, and fried foods. While many doctors recommend taking fat and caffeine out of the diet and increasing fiber, this has not been a satisfactory solution for most people. The low-FODMAP diet has been successful for some people.

It is still unclear to what extent diet causes the symptoms of IBS.

The Microbiome

The intestinal flora of IBS patients has been shown to differ from that of healthy controls, but the meaning of this is unclear since microbiota differ in many illnesses as well as between individuals.

Several studies have examined the role of the gut microbiota in IBS through manipulation with probiotics, antibiotics, fecal transplants, and germ-free animals. They have shown a relation between the microbiota and symptoms such as pain and bowel habits. Other studies are looking at the effect of stress on the intestinal microbiota. It continues to be an area of important research into possible therapeutic interventions for IBS.

Post-Infective IBS

> She was treated for parasites and we assumed she had knocked it out but wasn't well. Then she went to Central America and got amoebas and got treated. But she still wasn't feeling fantastic. One doctor told her it was all in her head. I was furious at this doctor. I don't think anybody wants to be sick. If you're sick, you're sick. If you're sick enough to complain about it, it's real.
>
> (ENID, 62)

A considerable number of cases of IBS are diagnosed following a GI infection. Patients get traveler's diarrhea, giardia (parasite infection), or campylobacter (food poisoning) and are never the same. (See chapter 14, "The Double Hit Theory.")

There are also cases of IBS following a diagnosis of inflammatory bowel disease (IBD). Illnesses such as IBD can cause more liquid to remain in the bowel, increasing the load of water that arrives in the large intestine and causing diarrhea. Excessive amounts of liquids in the bowel can also cause it to swell, and a red and inflamed gut can slow down the movement of the intestinal muscles, causing constipation. We also see many people with a diagnosis of celiac disease who respond well to a gluten-free diet and then appear to develop post-celiac IBS.

Brain-Gut Signal Problems

> I remember sitting in morning assembly in grade school just filled with pain.
>
> (ANNIE, 24)

It is said that IBS is "all in the head." Some is—the perception of pain is in the head—but the mechanism is in the gut.

Signals between the brain and the gut control how the intestines work. It is believed that disturbances in the neuroendocrine system that controls the motility (movement), secretions, and sensation within the gut may play a role in the development of IBS.

People with IBS have GI motor problems—i.e., slow or fast motility—that create spasms or sudden strong muscle contractions that can cause pain. And people with IBS have a lower pain threshold for the bowel stretching caused by gas or stool, leading to the hypothesis that their brain may process pain signals from the gut differently.

The "Gate" Theory of IBS

The Gate-Control Theory of pain perception suggests that the spinal cord contains a type of "gate" that opens and closes to allow or block pain signals traveling to the brain where they are interpreted and perceived.

It is proposed that people with IBS have gates that open more readily, and that the interpretation and perception of pain is amplified when they are experiencing psychological stress or distress. Pain is also a highly personal experience and difficult to measure. It can be influenced by expectations and augmented by psychological distress and strong emotions.

A maladaptive stress response may also contribute to the initiation, persistence, and severity of symptoms. Patients with IBS have a hyperreactivity or sensitivity to psychosocial factors such as a dramatic increase in bowel contraction in response to stress (e.g., final exams, presentations at work) or eating.

Psychological problems such as anxiety, depression, and PTSD are more common in people with IBS, although the link is unclear. GI disorders including IBS are often found in people who have reported past physical or sexual abuse. In a study we did of patients with celiac disease and persistent symptoms despite a strict gluten-free diet, a previous history of abuse (physical, emotional, or sexual) was shown to be the predominant driving factor of their symptoms.

Irritable bowel syndrome can be considered an example of the disruption of the complex relationships between the gut and the brain, and a better understanding of these alterations might provide new, targeted therapies. It is often addressed with psychological treatments, antidepressants, or both.

How Is IBS Treated?

We need to stop putting Band-Aids on symptoms and address the real problems behind common symptoms—such as bloating.

(FRAN, 69)

IBS is very difficult to treat. Most of the current medical options are limited to silencing symptoms but the more researchers uncover about the underlying causes of IBS, the more hope there is for drug therapies to treat them.

In addition, any one symptom can have a number of other diagnoses. Symptoms must be taken seriously even if the physician doesn't understand their mechanism of action.

Medications

The current arsenal for IBS medications includes:

- Laxatives for constipation
- Antidiarrheals to decrease the frequency of bowel movements
- Bile salt absorptive agents
- Antispasmodics to treat abdominal cramping and pain
- Antidepressants/psychotropics to treat pain and brain-gut dysfunction

The prescribing of antidepressants for IBS often elicits a response from patients of "You think this is all in my head!" or "I'm not depressed!" In fact, although antidepressants were developed to treat depression, they are also effective as analgesics, i.e., drugs that reduce pain. They block pain messages between the brain and the GI tract and reduce visceral hypersensitivity (within the inner organs). A recent study noted, "Much like treating diabetes with the insulin that is missing, antidepressants may help recover the brain's ability to respond to pain signals properly." Different categories of psychotropics also help treat diarrhea and constipation.

Antidepressants are often effective in treating IBS symptoms—we consider them "gut-otropics."

Serotonin

Serotonin, among its many activities, plays a major role in regulating peristalsis in the intestines as well as relaying sensory information to the brain. As noted in chapter 10 ("The 'Second Brain'"), mouse studies have demonstrated that *too little* serotonin can contribute to constipation, and *too much* can contribute to diarrhea. Studies are under way assessing abnormalities in serotonin transporters (SERT) as treatment in IBS. In addition, selective serotonin reuptake inhibitors (SSRIs) are a form of medication frequently prescribed for IBS.

Dietary Restriction

The majority of patients on a gluten-free diet have IBS and find the diet relieves some symptoms. What is unclear, however, is what aspects of wheat are causing their symptoms, whether this translates into an understanding or good treatment of the condition, and if it is an effective approach. It is clear that some people with diarrhea-predominant IBS (IBS-D) are wheat sensitive, and a trial of wheat or gluten restriction—after celiac disease has been excluded—is not unreasonable.

People with IBS often find relief with other types of dietary intervention such as lactose or fructose restriction. The low-FODMAP diet targets various carbohydrates (sugars) that are fermented in the colon by bacteria and create the gas and bloating characteristic of IBS. It is considered a miracle by some, and not truly effective by others.

Before commencing a strict FODMAP diet we would test for fructose intolerance. Fructose is a major component of the FODMAPs and, if positive, the avoidance of fructose-containing foods may be all that is required rather than the more restrictive FODMAP diet.

Probiotics

Probiotics are being studied as adjunctive therapy in treating IBS. To date, the studies have given researchers interesting observations, but the actual role of altered gut bacteria on the symptoms of IBS is unproven.

Supplements like probiotics are a largely unregulated market. Many contain unlabeled ingredients that may be harmful. (See chapter 5, "Supplements.") We suggest caution when taking various probiotics for IBS. Studies are often performed with products from specific manufacturers that may not be the same as those available over the counter.

Therapies for Mental Health Problems

Because cognitive processes play an important role in the top-down regulation of the body, various psychological treatments have been used to reduce pain and GI symptoms. This may include relaxation therapy or cognitive behavioral therapy to help modify the pain "gates" and stress responses in IBS.

Summary

- IBS is an extremely prevalent but poorly understood gastrointestinal disorder. While the gut can look normal, the disease is much more subtle pathologically.
- What we do understand is that it can interrupt everyday life with symptoms that are very real but whose causes are elusive.
- People with IBS appear to produce more gas in their GI tracts, eliminate it less effectively (promoting distension), and are more highly sensitized to the pain this causes. They also suffer from bouts of diarrhea and/or constipation—both often yo-yoing—triggered by a variety of environmental as well as physiological factors.
- Researchers are currently studying drugs that target diarrhea-predominant or constipation-predominant IBS.
- IBS is a condition that is often treated with dietary restrictions that may simply be a Band-Aid. As the science progresses, better therapies will become available. It is an area of intense research.

20

Inflammatory Bowel Disease

Most mornings I have a bout or two of diarrhea, and sometimes it
wakes me up at night. And it's liquid, just like a faucet. I can tell you,
it ain't no fun.

(GORDON, 52)

Inflammatory bowel disease (IBD) is the medical term for a digestive tract
on fire. And the inflammation in all or parts of the GI tract can ulcerate
and/or scar the intestines causing the pain, diarrhea, bleeding, and weight
loss common to the condition. The disease may be mild and restricted to
a localized area, or severe enough to require immunosuppressant drugs,
parenteral (intravenous) nutrition, or surgery.

While there is no one typical diet for people with IBD, dietary advice
and management are of great importance to patients with the disease.
Advice from the Internet or alternative medical practitioners is not a substitute for the role played by registered dietitians in the management of
disease activity, symptoms, and general nutrition.

What Is IBD?

My life revolves around it.

(BILL, 40)

IBD is the umbrella term for Crohn's disease, which may occur anywhere in the GI tract, and ulcerative colitis, which is limited to the colon. It is characterized by a recurring or chronically active inflammation originating in the intestines, but manifestations also occur outside of the tract. Some patients are classified as having intermediate colitis when it is not clear if they have Crohn's or colitis.

Colitis

Colitis is an inflammation of the colon. It may be mild, moderate, or severe, and is categorized by its causes. This includes infective (bacterial or viral), vascular (caused by a diminished blood supply to the colon), and immune based. The symptoms of colitis include diarrhea, cramping and pain, bleeding or bloody stools, *tenesmus* (the constant urge to have a bowel movement or sensation of incomplete evacuation), fever, fatigue, and other signs of inflammation.

Because some of these symptoms are also seen in IBS, celiac disease, and a number of other conditions, they are often confused, or mask a proper diagnosis.

Crohn's Disease

Crohn's disease can affect the entire GI tract—from the mouth to the anus—not just the colon. The symptoms are similar to other inflammatory bowel diseases, but abdominal pain is usually more prominent and bleeding less prominent than in ulcerative colitis.

It is important that you seek medical help if the diarrhea is persistent or you become dehydrated. Fever and blood in the stool are alarm symptoms that require an aggressive diagnostic approach.

What Causes IBD?

Stress and diet were once believed to initiate IBD, but it is now understood that they only aggravate the symptoms. Because inflammation can be ascertained through tests, we understand a lot about the gut itself in diseases like IBD, but uncovering its causes has proven more difficult.

IBD is a complex disease that appears to occur due to a combination of:

- genes
- an inappropriate immune response in the gut triggers inflammation
- the microbiome
- environmental factors

Recent studies are beginning to connect some of the dots.

Genes

Genes appear to be a factor, as the condition is found in clusters in some families. Ten to 20 percent of people with IBD have a family history of the disease. Thus, the genetic influence on microbial content in the gut is also thought to play a role.

Immune Responses

One theory regarding the development of IBD involves an inappropriate immune response within the gut that creates inflammation. It is thought that this response is triggered by a disturbed tolerance to antigens (toxins, bacteria) found in the *lumen*. And most of these antigens are derived from the intestinal microbiota.

The Microbiome

The colonization of the intestine by microbes in early life is the main stimulus that matures the immune system in babies. (See chapter 9, "The Microbiome.") This is an active and fluid process that depends on genetic and environmental factors.

Scientists are beginning to explore the possibility that the composition of our intestinal microbiota could contribute to inflammatory conditions in the gut. In people whose microbiota respond inappropriately to what is going through the digestive tract, the normal low-grade inflammation that keeps us safe from pathogens goes into overdrive and starts to damage and/or destroy the mucosal lining. There may be a similar genetic/microbiotic/environmental storm at work in celiac disease.

Studies on the microbiotic makeup of patients with IBD are being conducted. One study showed that people with IBD had 30 to 50 percent reduced biodiversity in *Firmicutes* and *Bacteroidetes,* two of the major classes of bacteria populating the gut. The Firmicutes family includes many "friendly" bacteria that are essential for digestion and balance in the body and others such as *Streptococcus* and *Clostridium* that cause infections when they overgrow.

Further evidence of the role of gut flora in the cause of inflammatory bowel disease is that affected individuals are more likely to have been prescribed antibiotics in the two- to five-year period before their diagnosis than unaffected individuals. The microbiome can be altered by environmental factors such as food or oral medications—antibiotics, iron preparations—but no direct link to specific diseases has been proven.

Future studies are necessary to determine the meaning of the complex interactions between our gut and our microbiota and the respective role each plays in inflammatory diseases such as IBD.

Environmental Factors

A number of environmental factors have been implicated in IBD. They include:

- **Geography:** The disease has concentrations in certain parts of the U.S. and the world
- **Smoking:** For unknown reasons smokers are at lower risk of developing ulcerative colitis while Crohn's disease is more common among smokers.
- **Medications:** Antibiotics and NSAIDs may aggravate symptoms rather than cause them, yet they have been implicated in the condition.

The Western diet—with its low-fiber, high-fat, and high-sugar content—has been implicated in the development of IBD, but there is little evidence to back up this supposition. Advice about anti-inflammatory, Paleo, low-carb, specific carbohydrate, or gluten-free diets abounds. However, they have not been studied and may place unnecessary nutritional burdens on patients with IBD.

Liquid diets have been studied in the dietary manipulation of Crohn's disease with some interesting results regarding the relation of food to the causes of IBD. The exclusive or partial enteral nutrition diets replace foods with predigested liquid. Gluten, animal fat, and dairy products are among the restricted items on these diets. The response to these dietary therapies in terms of remission rates is high—equivalent to the response to steroid therapy, a mainstay of treatment for IBD. While the mechanism remains unclear, it has moved from the concept of "bowel rest" to hypotheses about the effects on the intestinal microbiome, intestinal barrier repair, and the immune system. The dramatic response rate to the lack of specific foods and the presence of predigested dietary components highlight the role of food or specific components of food in the genesis—and possible treatment—of this disease.

How Is IBD Diagnosed?

They went in from the top and they went in from the bottom. The doctor showed me a picture—which meant little to me—of these fissures and said, "This is abnormal."

(GORDON, 52)

IBD is diagnosed through a variety of tests that may include endoscopy and/or colonoscopy with biopsy, blood and stool tests, and X-rays or scans in order to determine if the GI tract is inflamed and injured, as well as the extent and location of the damage. A patient history of symptoms and frequency and what environmental or dietary factors affect them is also taken.

How Is IBD Treated?

Treatment for IBD will depend on whether a patient has Crohn's disease or some form of colitis. It is usually some combination of medications to reduce inflammation, induce healing, and relieve symptoms, and/or surgery.

Diet

Dietary advice is essential in IBD. Since the inflammation of the GI tract can cause the malabsorption of essential vitamins and minerals leading to malnutrition, these deficiencies must be addressed. Nutrient deficiencies including vitamin B12, iron, vitamin D, and folic acid can be measured and treated when necessary.

After bouts of diarrhea, it is also important for patients to replenish lost water.

There are restriction diets used to control symptoms, and they vary with a patient's diagnosis, food intolerances, and other conditions that may occur simultaneously. Up to one-third of patients continue to have symptoms in the absence of inflammatory disease activity. This may be post–IBD irritable bowel syndrome, or a functional disorder caused by a fructose or FODMAP sensitivity that needs to be determined.

Lactose intolerance is common in ulcerative colitis, so avoiding milk products will alleviate symptoms for these people. Reducing fiber or specific foods that trigger symptoms often helps people who have flares or strictures.

Celiac Disease, Gluten, and IBD

My colitis improved since I started a gluten-free diet! Do I have celiac disease?

(WAYNE, 50)

On one hand, celiac disease and IBD can occur together, but the improvement may coincide with a remission in the IBD, since the disease is subject to spontaneous flares and remissions. In addition, the improvement of symptoms on a gluten-free diet may be due to the reduction of other carbohydrates. All of this highlights the need to be tested for celiac disease before starting a gluten-free diet.

Celiac disease does occur more commonly in IBD patients than in the general population. It is important to note that people can have two diseases and/or other food intolerances.

Summary

- IBD is a complex group of conditions that inflame and ulcerate the bowel. It requires an accurate medical diagnosis and dietary treatment.
- If you do go on an elimination diet, seek the help of a registered dietitian. There is evidence that a significant number of IBD patients are reducing gluten. Whether this alleviates symptoms is unclear, as is the effectiveness of the currently popular "anti-inflammatory" diets. There is no evidence that either diet actually reduces the inflammatory response causing the disease in the gut.
- It is especially important to remember that the symptoms of IBD overlap with those of other conditions and food intolerances.
- This is an area where isolating the issue, testing, and only then treating is particularly relevant.

21

Eosinophilic Esophagitis

A good listener is a good talker with a sore throat.
—KATHERINE WHITEHORN

Eosinophilic esophagitis (EoE) is an emerging food-related disorder. It is a specific type of inflammation of the esophagus that may cause food to become stuck in this muscular tube that connects the mouth to the stomach. It is seen in children as well as adults. Unlike other GI conditions such as celiac disease or IBS, it affects men more than women.

People often minimize symptoms, feeling that they will go away, are caused by eating too quickly, or are something the individual can live with. Children with the condition are often told that they are not chewing their food well or are eating too quickly. A lack of awareness of the condition in the medical community means that symptoms are often overlooked or misdiagnosed.

What Is EoE?

EoE is an inflammation of the esophagus characterized by dysfunction in the esophagus and the presence of eosinophils (white blood cells associated with allergies) in the mucosal tissue lining the esophagus. Patients typically complain of food "sticking" in the throat, although this symptom is not always present.

Other symptoms include:

- difficulty or pain with swallowing
- food becoming lodged within the esophagus
- refusal to eat or failure to thrive in children
- vomiting with meals
- heartburn

EoE may also coexist with other GI conditions, including celiac disease. Celiac disease and EoE are both associated with an aberrant immune response to food antigens and the different studies have demonstrated an association between the two. This is interesting, as the nature of the immune response is different in the two conditions. But both require endoscopy for diagnosis.

What Causes EoE?

There are two types of EoE. The main cause is an allergic immune response to specific foods. Because some people respond to intensive treatment for gastrointestinal reflux disease (GERD), we are aware that reflux may cause EoE. Esophagitis—an inflammation of the esophagus—is also caused by a number of other mechanisms including infections (viral and fungal) and radiation therapy. This is different from a diagnosis of EoE.

Food Allergy

The leading theory about the cause of eosinophilic esophagitis is that it represents a food allergy. The hallmark is the presence of a large number of eosinophils, a white blood cell associated with other allergic conditions, in the wall of the esophagus. Studies using elimination diets have shown a reversal of the esophagitis and disappearance of the eosinophils confirming this mechanism.

GERD

Some patients suffering from EoE have GERD, which is much more common, and will see symptoms resolved with medications, typically proton pump inhibitors (PPIs). (See chapter 8, "The Gut in Disease.") After a diagnosis of EoE, a trial of high-dose PPIs is often undertaken to assess if that will resolve symptoms and normalize biopsy results.

Interestingly, the pathological features of EoE due to GERD are similar to that of EoE caused by a food allergy. Pathologists examining biopsies of patients with GERD sometimes find "nests" of eosinophils.

Diagnosis of EoE

The diagnosis of eosinophilic esophagitis is done during an endoscopy. Biopsies then confirm the presence of a great number of eosinophils.

The tests for food allergies in EoE are not considered reliable. These include blood tests for IgE antibodies to specific foods and skin or patch tests. The most reliable tests are elimination diets in which people are advised to go on an exclusion diet eliminating the eight major food groups known to cause allergic reactions (dairy, soy, peanuts, tree nuts, eggs, wheat, fish, and shellfish). Different categories are then added back one by one until the offending food is found.

Often multiple endoscopies are performed to assess the effect of withdrawal, and foods are reintroduced based on the findings.

Treatment

The treatment for EoE depends on the age of the patient and the severity of symptoms. Swallowed steroids are the mainstay of treatment for symptom relief. Inhalers of the type used in the treatment of asthma are prescribed, with patients instructed to swallow, not inhale, the drug.

Patients with a markedly narrow esophagus may require stretching or dilation. This is done with some apprehension, however, as in some cases this can rupture the esophagus.

Summary

EoE is a disease that has become more prevalent in the past decade. It is primarily a food-related sensitivity.

Like celiac disease, other allergies, and autoimmune conditions, it is on the rise. This raises the intriguing question—what are the environmental triggers responsible for this remarkable change in medicine in the past few decades?

22

Neuropathy

Science is wonderfully equipped to answer the question "How?"
but it gets terribly confused when you ask the question "Why?"
—ERWIN CHARGAFF

I found out about peripheral neuropathy because I'm old-fashioned.
You see, I still write checks. I couldn't hold the pen to sign my name.
And when I did, it didn't look like my signature. My kids told me it
was time to switch to online banking, but I figured it was time to
see a doctor.

(LILA, 59)

The nervous system and brain are perhaps the most complex and elusive
parts of the human body. Nerve fibers run to, from, and through every
inch of our frame—we are, quite literally, a bundle of nerves. Compound-
ing this is the "second brain" in our gut that has a mind and plenty of
"nerve" of its own. (See chapter 10.)

The nervous system is the regulator and monitor of every organ and
system in the body and is intimately involved in our perception of the
world. It is at once the wise and benign sovereign of all movement, coordination, and sensation, and the devil-like source of all pain.

Recently there have been claims that gluten is destroying our brains—a
dangerously simplistic approach to an intricate system that is difficult to
visualize and whose mechanisms are still largely unknown. While science
has a good grasp of how the nervous system functions, the mechanisms

behind and treatment of its malfunctions currently offer more questions than answers.

Gluten may actually play a role in nervous system malfunctions such as the neuropathies and ataxias suffered by some, but removing it from your diet is not a cure and may not even be an effective treatment.

What Is a Neuropathy?

The word *neuropathy* (*neuro,* "nervous system"; *pathy,* "disease of") encompasses all the nerves in the body. This includes:

- autonomic nerves (that control involuntary or unconscious nerves)
- motor nerves (that control movement of limbs, etc.)
- sensory nerves (that transmit various information about hot, cold, pain, position)

A person's symptoms depend on the type of neuropathy and the type of nerves affected. Our focus will be on the peripheral neuropathies and ataxia that appear to be related to gluten.

Peripheral Neuropathy

Try holding chopsticks when your fingers are numb.

(RITA, 36)

Peripheral neuropathies are a general term to explain an alteration of normal sensation occurring usually in the hands, feet, and face. They create *paresthesia* (a burning or tingling), as well as numbness, cramps, restless legs, and especially pain in the hands and feet, and sometimes other parts of the body.

Most people have experienced paresthesia—a feeling of pins and needles—at some time in their lives. When you sit with crossed legs for too long, a leg may fall asleep. This occurs because sustained pressure is placed on a nerve; the leg "wakes up" once the pressure is relieved. The paresthesia may be mild or severe enough to interfere with normal function and activities.

Chronic *neuropathies* are often a symptom of an underlying neurological disease or traumatic nerve damage. While diabetes is the most common cause of neuropathy, other medical conditions can also lead to the problem; these include vitamin or mineral deficiencies, Lyme disease, inflammation, trauma, excessive alcohol intake, Guillain-Barré syndrome, infections, pressure on nerves (computer use or sports related), celiac disease, and various pharmaceuticals.

Diabetic Neuropathy

Most cases of neuropathy are found in people who have type 1 diabetes, though it also occurs in type 2 diabetics. Diabetic neuropathy is a microvascular (involving small blood vessels) complication of the disease. Elevated levels of blood sugar in people with diabetes can, over time, injure the walls of the tiny blood vessels that supply nerves. Since one consequence of the nerve damage can be an inability to feel pain, problems can go unnoticed until digits are badly injured, especially in the legs. In the U.S., 50 to 70 percent of people with diabetes have some form of diabetic neuropathy. A diabetic patient's neuropathy often affects the gut (autonomic neuropathy), causing *gastroparesis*.

Autoimmune Disease and Neuropathy

Neuropathies are common in various other autoimmune diseases. The neuropathies found in celiac disease appear to be related to vitamin deficiencies, inflammation, and/or autoimmune factors. Symptoms consistent with neuropathy are common when people are diagnosed, and often disappear on a gluten-free diet. We routinely test patients with celiac disease and neuropathy for vitamin deficiencies (see page 212).

People with nonceliac gluten sensitivity (NCGS) may also feel that these symptoms resolve when gluten is removed. Yet some patients on a gluten-free diet develop peripheral neuropathies at a later date. This may be due to the development of a new autoimmune disease or as a result of the gluten-free diet itself—a heavy-metal toxicity (lead, mercury, arsenic) or a B vitamin deficiency. (See chapter 4, "Perils of a Gluten-Free Diet.")

Ataxia

When I went to an ataxia patient meeting, I wasn't prepared for what I saw. I encountered many people who struggled with or were unable to perform daily tasks that we take for granted, like walking, cutting their steak, or having a glass of water.

(ARMIN ALAEDINI, PH.D., BIOCHEMIST AND IMMUNOLOGIST)

Ataxia creates problems with balance, movement, and coordination. It describes a lack of muscle control during voluntary movements, such as walking or picking up objects. Ataxia can affect movement, speech, eye movement, and swallowing. It is also associated with degenerative diseases of the central nervous system. Persistent ataxia usually results from damage to your cerebellum—the part of your brain that controls muscle coordination. It is also seen in people with neuropathies because of an altered perception of the position of their limbs.

Many conditions can cause ataxia, including alcohol abuse, stroke, tumor, cerebral palsy, and multiple sclerosis. Inherited defective genes also can cause ataxia. About 40 percent of ataxias are genetic, but 60 percent are idiopathic (of unknown origin). In various studies, 9 to 15 percent of patients with idiopathic ataxia have celiac disease. In fact, some researchers believe that as many as 40 percent of the cases of idiopathic ataxia are gluten related.

Gluten Ataxia

Gluten ataxia (GA) is defined as an ataxia where other underlying causes cannot be ascertained and antigliadin antibodies are present. It is associated with cerebellar atrophy, where cells in the area of the brain controlling coordination and balance deteriorate and die. Some research indicates that GA may be immune mediated and part of the spectrum of gluten sensitivity, but this is open to question.

In a UK study, 40 percent of sporadic ataxia patients were positive for IgG antibodies to gluten. But the meaning of the presence of antigliadin antibodies in these patients is not fully understood. These are nonceliac antibodies also found in a percentage of people with a number of conditions, including ADHD and autism. The presence of these antibodies must be shown to have a direct effect on function to be considered significant.

At this point, the direct pathological effect on neural function of antigliadin antibodies is still being debated. If it is possible to eliminate these antibodies through a strict gluten-free diet, it may have important therapeutic implications, though this has not been demonstrated. (See chapter 6, "Testing—What Do Antibodies Tell Us?")

Researchers in Finland and England have studied the brains of people with gluten ataxia and found deposits of gluten antibodies around blood vessels in their brains. These investigators also found antibodies in the brain to transglutaminase 6 (TG6), a form of TG2, the enzyme that reacts with gliadin and sets off the reaction that triggers celiac disease. They feel these individuals develop antibodies to TG6 in an immune response to gluten. These results need to be duplicated by other researchers before the development of a test for GA will be commercially available.

Nevertheless, it is an intriguing finding that may uncover one of the few treatable causes of idiopathic sporadic ataxia.

There is also interest in the potential for an individual's immune response to gluten to cross-react with certain proteins found in the brain such as *synapsin I*. Synapsin I is a complex protein that does many things in the body, especially in the nervous system. In simple terms, it can act as a "shuttle" that helps in the transmission of nerve signals. As Armin Alaedini, a biochemist and immunologist at Columbia University, explains, "We have shown that antibodies to gliadin can cross-react and bind to the synapsin I protein. This does not necessarily mean that such cross-reactivity will cause neurologic disease but if the antibodies can access and bind to the protein, they may interfere with its functions or create a harmful inflammatory response against nerve tissue."

These findings open a window into the potential effect of the immune response to gluten on the nervous system. This may lead to an understanding of the mechanisms beneath the neurological symptoms found in gluten sensitivity; and the role that antibodies to gliadin may play in modifying cellular signaling within the nervous system.

How Is Neuropathy Diagnosed?

Peripheral neuropathies are diagnosed by a physical examination and patient history, as well as *nerve conduction studies* (EMG) and laboratory tests. The small-fiber neuropathies associated with celiac disease are not the larger nerves tested in EMG. Therefore these EMG studies will be normal in people with celiac disease who have a peripheral neuropathy. Instead, we perform a skin biopsy that is stained to highlight the small nerve fibers. The diagnosis is made when the small nerve fibers are seen to be absent or reduced.

Ataxias are diagnosed based on a person's medical history, family history, and a complete neurological evaluation, including an MRI scan of the brain to determine if there is damage. Various blood tests may be performed to rule out other possible disorders that may present similar symptoms. Genetic testing is also available to determine if the ataxia is inherited.

Vitamin deficiencies (E, B12, B1, B2, and B6) and copper deficiency need to be excluded, as well as vitamin B6 toxicity.

How Is Neuropathy Treated?

The appropriate treatment for neuropathy depends on accurate diagnosis of the underlying cause. And since this is often unclear, most treatments focus on symptom relief.

For peripheral neuropathies, therapies such as electrical nerve stimulation, physical therapy, surgery to release compressed nerves, and various medications can resolve symptoms for many. Drugs such as IV gamma globulin and NSAIDs can be helpful. Frequently, SSRIs are prescribed.

There is conflicting data on the effect of a gluten-free diet. Putting the majority of the blame on gluten is a mistake, and even in people with celiac disease, a gluten-free diet does not always resolve symptoms. Some people see a complete reversal of symptoms, others find the symptoms are less severe, and some develop peripheral neuropathies while on a gluten-free diet. Others improve through nutritional supplementation because they are mal-absorbing the B vitamins, minerals, or other trace elements.

Summary

- Neuropathy is the result of a number of underlying medical conditions. It often exists without a clear cause—what doctors classify as idiopathic, of unknown origin.
- Peripheral neuropathies are fairly common. Everyone, at some point in his or her life, will probably have some type of neuro-

logical symptom. They are associated with a number of diseases and lifestyles. Recently, the science of ergonomics developed, to prevent musculoskeletal disorders in the workplace—which often includes paresthesia of the hands, wrists, back, and arms from computer use.

- Ataxia is a rare disease but disrupts function for those with the condition. It can be mild—occasional loss of balance—or paralyzing. In the absence of celiac disease, the presence of antigliadin antibodies indicates a gluten connection in some people.

- The cross-reaction of gluten with proteins in the brain is being studied in various neurological conditions. At this point, the mechanisms behind various neurological complications in gluten-related disorders are not clear.

- While gluten may be a cause of both neuropathy and ataxia, numerous other conditions need to be excluded before adopting a gluten-free diet.

Nevertheless, studies linking gluten to various neuropathies provide a tantalizing link between the gut and the brain.

23

Diabetes

You always have diabetes. Every moment you have diabetes. It's either something you're consciously thinking of, or it's there and you're going to have to think about it. *Is my blood sugar high, is it low? When do I have to eat? Or should I eat?*

Being on an insulin pump has made an enormous difference in that, but the potential for something getting out of control is there.

(ART, 67)

In the U.S. today, there are approximately 21 million people who have been diagnosed with diabetes. About 1.25 million of them have type 1 or insulin-dependent diabetes mellitus (IDDM). In the UK, approximately 3.2 million people have diabetes and the number is estimated by Diabetes UK to rise to 5 million by 2025. Studies show that about 10 percent of this group will also develop celiac disease. However, the role that gluten may play in the development of IDDM is a new and intriguing finding in the search for the mechanisms leading to this disease and the search for a cure.

There is a recognized association between celiac disease and type 1 or IDDM. The same association does not exist with type 2. Many clinics screen diabetic children for celiac disease, although the symptoms are often silent or go unrecognized. In fact, many doctors and clinics view the "double diagnosis" as a huge burden and will not test unless pushed by parents or the development of symptoms. This may not be a wise choice.

What Is Diabetes?

In the middle of final exams during my senior year in college, I started to have strange physical symptoms. I was experiencing extreme thirst and very frequent urination, always getting up in the middle of the night to go to the bathroom. Initially, my friends and I joked about it—"What the hell is this?" In response to the thirst, I would—in retrospect, absurdly—drink a bunch of sugared soda to quench my thirst, and then go to the bathroom even more. And it finally reached a point where I said, "I better go and do something about this." I went to the university medical clinic and was diagnosed with what is now called type 1 diabetes. That was forty-seven years ago.

(ART, 67)

Diabetes mellitus (from the Greek for "go through" and "sweet") describes a lack or deficiency of insulin, a hormone that enables the body to metabolize and use glucose (sugar). Glucose is a fuel that is critical for muscle, brain, and body function. Unable to enter the cells, it accumulates in the blood until it gets to the kidneys, where fluid is drawn from the body in order to excrete the excess sugar, which then spills into the urine. This causes the thirst and frequent glucose-filled urination Art describes, and a recognized symptom of the disease.

If the diabetes is not corrected, the body becomes starved for energy and begins drawing on fat and protein stores, leading to weight loss and muscle wasting. This emergency process releases fatty acids (in the form of ketones) into the bloodstream, which can lead to coma or death.

There are two types of diabetes.

Type 1, or insulin-dependent diabetes mellitus (IDDM), formerly referred to as juvenile-onset diabetes, is an autoimmune disorder that occurs mainly in younger people, but can occur in adults. The immune system attacks and destroys the pancreatic islets where the insulin-producing cells reside, setting off the sequence of events described on page 215. When insulin is no longer produced by the body, it must be permanently replaced by injections/pump.

Type 2, or non-insulin-dependent diabetes mellitus (NIDDM), so-called adult onset diabetes, appears to start as an insulin resistance, a condition in which the insulin produced is less effective in controlling blood glucose. Type 2 diabetes is not an autoimmune condition, and insulin production is unstable, not absent. The condition appears to have a genetic or family association and occurs more commonly in people with obesity and older age. However, it is increasingly being seen in overweight children whose cells cannot handle the amount of carbohydrates they are consuming.

Type 2 diabetics can often control their condition through diet alone or with oral (non-insulin) medications. Some will also require insulin shots to control blood glucose levels.

A third type, *gestational diabetes*, occurs during pregnancy and is usually temporary. The mother's body does not respond to insulin, and the condition can normally be controlled with diet alone. The condition usually resolves itself once the baby is born.

What Causes Diabetes?

The destruction of the islet cells of the pancreas, which produce insulin, in IDDM appears to be caused by several factors. While the precise trigger is not clear, it is believed to include an autoimmune reaction, infections that attack the islet cells, and other environmental factors that initiate the autoimmune process. The possible role of the microbiome is also of emerging interest.

Is Gluten a Trigger in IDDM?

Celiac disease is 5 to 7 percent more common in people with IDDM than in the general population. It is not more common in people with NIDDM.

There is evidence that patients diagnosed with celiac disease later in life have a higher rate of IDDM than patients diagnosed at a younger age. This indicates that a longer exposure to gluten increases the risk of developing IDDM in susceptible individuals.

Furthermore, two large human studies established an association between an early infant diet containing gluten and the development of autoantibodies (antibodies against "self") against the islet cells.

Several animal studies have documented that the development of IDDM is influenced by diet. While a gluten-free diet largely prevented the onset of diabetes in one study of mice specially bred with a susceptibility to develop IDDM, the mechanisms underlying the influence of gluten on the incidence of IDDM in humans are not fully understood.

Some studies have shown that gluten creates an inflammatory response affecting the microbiota. It raises the feasibility of early dietary interventions for IDDM and the need to determine if and how dietary intervention can affect immune regulation and disease development.

Diabetes and the Microbiome

The microbiome plays an important role in shaping immune responses in the gut as well as in the development of autoimmunity. A growing number of human studies demonstrate differences in the microbiome of people with IDDM versus controls. This supports the idea that alterations in the microbiome precede the onset of IDDM. Since the microbiome is sculpted and remodeled extensively in the first few years of life, there may be a window of opportunity to modify risk factors in children who have markers of anti-islet autoimmunity.

Studies are looking to find the mechanism(s), timeline, and possible therapeutic options to prevent the disease by altering the microbiome.

The Dual Diagnosis

As mentioned earlier, approximately 10 percent of all diabetics have a double diagnosis of celiac disease and IDDM. The link to gluten exposure as a potential triggering factor of the autoimmune reaction gives further validity to the need to test children with IDDM for celiac disease.

This raises the question of whether all children with IDDM should be routinely screened. A recent study showed tremendous variability on this question, as well as in the guidelines of different authoritative groups regarding which tests to use and the timing and frequency of those tests.

The Pros for Screening

There are several well-defined links between celiac disease and diabetes. Both are associated with similar *HLA (human leukocyte antigen) genes*. They are both autoimmune diseases where autoantibodies are present in children. Having one autoimmune disease increases the risk of getting another.

Those who advocate routine screening emphasize that patients with IDDM may have no symptoms or silent symptoms that are only recognized retrospectively. In addition, there are complications of untreated celiac disease, and it is better to pick up the potential subtle changes that might affect learning and achievement.

Symptoms to look for include:

- GI complaints, common in both diseases, should not be overlooked; mild symptoms such as bloating are often recognized retrospectively

- growth issues (failure to thrive)
- delayed puberty
- anemia
- fatigue
- iron deficiency
- dental enamel defects
- hypoglycemia and a reduction in insulin requirements, or "ping-ponging" when food is not being absorbed
- vitamin/mineral deficiencies
- elevated liver enzymes

Interestingly, in a recent study in the *Diabetes Educator,* 49 percent of the respondents to a screening test reported that their patients improved with a gluten-free diet despite not being aware of symptoms prior to the diagnosis of celiac disease. It is unclear what percentage of physicians test for celiac disease in diabetic patients.

The Cons

Some argue against routine screening, claiming that it can affect quality of life, and that the outcome of subclinical celiac disease in diabetes is not fully investigated. Evidence is inconclusive as to whether the benefits of screening and potentially treating asymptomatic individuals outweigh the harms of managing a population already burdened with a serious illness.

Nevertheless, we recommend testing people with IDDM for celiac disease because of the high prevalence and the potential benefits of treatment with a gluten-free diet. This includes control of symptoms, stabilization of diabetes, and prevention of complications associated with celiac disease.

Recent population-based studies following patients with both IDDM and celiac disease for nearly 40 years showed a significantly higher mortality for these people than those who just had celiac disease. This implies that undiagnosed celiac disease is not a benign condition and needs to be diagnosed and treated. The explanation for the increased risk of death included:

- persistent low-grade inflammation due to disease activity
- poor adherence to the gluten-free diet
- difficulty following a gluten-free diet and insulin therapy

This study also highlights the need for excellence in both the care of the diabetes and of the celiac disease.

Treating the Double Diagnosis—Glucose and Gluten

A lot of these children are on the pump for a few years, are well managed and coping, and then [are] told "you have to be gluten-free." They did not necessarily feel bad to begin with, are already "different," and don't want to be gluten-free. Some manage it really well, and others don't. My goal is to encourage them to consider being gluten-free and to do so in a healthy way.

(SUZANNE SIMPSON, R.D.)

Our daughter was diagnosed with type 1 diabetes when she turned 4 and celiac disease two weeks afterward. From our perspective the celiac is more difficult to deal with. There's not much that she can't eat in relation to type 1 as long as we prepare and plan ahead, and cover her with the right amount of insulin. In terms of celiac disease, she needs to be totally gluten-free, and we're finding that a huge challenge.

(RAY, 38)

Most people with IDDM receive the diabetes diagnosis first and they develop the skills, knowledge, and how-to to manage the diabetes and blood sugar and insulin. And then they get diagnosed with celiac disease and many say it is harder having celiac disease than diabetes. On one hand, this may be due to having mastered the care of their diabetes—you can adjust your insulin to compensate for the candy bar you want—but with celiac disease you cannot just "take something" if you want to eat gluten or think you have inadvertently eaten it. It also means rethinking glucose in terms of its high presence in gluten-free foods.

Treating people with type 1 diabetes and celiac disease involves mind as well as matter. Balancing diet, lifestyle, and compliance is like walking an emotional and physical tightrope and can be difficult. Many do not have gastrointestinal symptoms, so the motivation to be gluten-free is not high.

> The hardest part is not getting a break—it is sort of a double whammy of having to think about your food from two different perspectives. You have two conditions and you have to think about them all the time.
>
> (SUZANNE SIMPSON, R.D.)

Carbohydrates from Two Perspectives

Dietary management in diabetes is based on controlling blood sugar levels. It is a combination of food, exercise/lifestyle, and insulin. When you look at food as a diabetic, you are looking primarily at the carbohydrates, since insulin regulation is based on the amount of carbohydrates in the food and your blood sugar levels at that particular moment.

When you have celiac disease, you are also focused on food—specifically gluten. And gluten-free foods are usually much higher in starch/carbohydrates, lower in fiber than their wheat-based counterparts, and have a different impact on blood sugar. The glycemic response to many gluten-free foods varies from patient to patient, but tends to be higher and faster. It is also important to be aware of the inadequacies of a gluten-free diet. (See chapter 4, "Pitfalls and Perils of a Gluten-Free Diet.")

The balance of food, insulin, and level of activity takes on an added dimension that must be learned and integrated into a lifestyle. This can be particularly hard on adolescents who live—and tend to enjoy—more spontaneous and unpredictable lives. Planning often means "let's go!"

> The biggest thing for me is that I'm concerned that she's losing a bit of her childhood in a way, being forced to think about things a 4-year-old wouldn't have to face. I wonder how that's going to affect her. It seems that there's sort of a loss of innocence I feel bad about.
>
> (RAY, 38)

Children and adolescents with a double diagnosis must buy into their own care. This may require the assistance not only of parents, but dietitians they trust and support groups that offer peer assistance. A sharing support system of family and friends is essential.

Despite the psychological burdens of a dual glucose- and gluten-restricted diet, the price paid for noncompliance is very high. Patients must learn to embrace a "live with" rather than "life without" lifestyle.

Summary

- The role(s) of gluten in the development of IDDM via its effect on autoimmune and inflammatory processes and the microbiome are being actively studied. They may offer an exciting pathway to block the development of IDDM.
- Is there a "switch" at play? If so, is there a time frame for turning it off or ensuring that it is not turned on?
- A gluten-free diet will not cure someone already diagnosed with type 1 diabetes or reverse any of its complications. Studies indicate that antigliadin antibodies do disappear on a gluten-free diet, and this may have a positive effect on those with a dual diagnosis, especially children.

24

Wheat and Other
Food Allergies

In Candy Land there are a few things that can happen to you when you get to jump across the board. One is getting a lollipop and one is getting a peppermint candy and one is getting a peanut. And [my granddaughter] drew the peanut, and she said, "Eek! I can't have peanuts, get it away from me." I told her that her playing piece could jump on that square but that she wouldn't really eat it. We don't put the whole Candy Land away just because it has a peanut.

(MARY, 67)

Food allergies are a potentially lethal cousin of a food intolerance or sensitivity. While many people avoid wheat because it makes them bloated, gassy, or fatigued, others must avoid wheat because it makes their throats swell and breathing increasingly difficult and sometimes impossible.

Food allergies are one of the most common medical disorders and affect up to 15 million Americans and more than 17 million in Europe. A study by the CDC showed that food allergies increased by about 50 percent between 1997 and 2011. The upsurge in allergies is part of the medical puzzle surrounding our unexpected and increasing reactions to various foods.

What Are Food Allergies?

Food allergies are caused when your immune system sees an otherwise harmless food or substance as an invader (allergen). It releases antibodies, specifically IgE antibodies, to neutralize the perceived threat. These are different from the IgA and IgG antibodies seen in food intolerances and sensitivities. (See chapter 6, "Antibodies.") The first encounter is usually benign and simply sensitizes that person to the food. But when the IgE antibodies "see" that antigen again, they trigger the release of chemicals such as *histamines*, causing the symptoms that characterize an allergic reaction. This may include swelling, itching, hives, asthma, vomiting, diarrhea, respiratory distress, and shock. The reactions range from mild—itchy skin or mouth—to severe *anaphylaxis*, which can be life threatening.

IgE allergic reactions are immediate, usually occurring within seconds or up to several hours, and involve the whole body. They are different from the delayed sensitivity described in previous chapters. Allergens can be to different foods, drugs, insect bites and stings, as well as pollens, mold spores, animal dander, and dust mites.

They directly affect a person's quality of life and require extreme vigilance when eating out or traveling. Most children will outgrow allergies to eggs, dairy, wheat, and soy, possibly because of the immune system's response to the food. Allergies to peanuts, seafood, and tree nuts are rarely lost.

Specific Food-Induced Allergies

> There was one kiwi slice on top of the fruit salad, so I thought I'd just dig underneath. That was hospital trip number one.
>
> (GEORGE, 19)

There are eight categories of major food allergens (the so-called Big 8)—milk, eggs, fish, shellfish, tree nuts, peanuts, wheat, and soybeans. The

USA Food Allergen Labeling Act requires that they must be listed on all processed food labels. These foods account for about 90 percent of all food allergies, but people can also be allergic to various seeds, legumes (including peanuts and soybeans), fruits, corn, vegetables, and various herbs and spices.

Allergies also occur in conjunction with other conditions, such as asthma, and in certain professions, i.e., baker's asthma.

Allergic Asthma

Allergies and asthma can occur together. Asthma is a lung disease that causes the airways to become inflamed and narrowed. It occurs often in childhood and its causes are unclear, but appear to have both genetic and environmental origins. For many people, it is connected to an allergic reaction to a specific food or substance. Over 50 percent of people suffering from asthma have allergic asthma. While many of these reactions are directed against dust, pollen, and airborne substances, several are food related.

Children who have food allergies as well as asthma are at an increased risk for a more severe reaction to both. The relationship between the two does not appear to be causal. It is crucial that patients are educated about avoiding the offending food(s) and the emergency use of asthma and allergy medications in the event of a reaction.

Baker's Asthma

Baker's asthma is the most common cause of occupational asthma, and annual incidences of the disease range between 1 and 10 cases per 1,000 bakery workers. The main agents that cause baker's asthma are cereal flours (wheat, rye, and barley) and enzymes. Baker's asthma is IgE mediated and can affect anyone working in a bakery, confectionery, flour miller, and/or food processing facility.

Wheat-Dependent
Exercise-Induced Anaphylaxis

Wheat-dependent exercise-induced anaphylaxis (WDEIA) is a rare disorder where exercise that occurs after ingesting an allergen triggers anaphylaxis. This can occur even though the exercise and allergen exposure are tolerated independently of each other. It is one clinical form of IgE-mediated allergy to wheat. Wheat is not the only food associated with food-exercise-induced anaphylaxis—it was first described with celery!

Eosinophilic Esophagitis

Eosinophilic esophagitis is an allergic reaction to food that causes swelling of the tissue in the esophagus. (For a fuller description, see chapter 21, "Eosinophilic Esophagitis.")

What Causes Food Allergies?

When my granddaughter was a few weeks old, they noticed blood in her diaper. So the pediatrician said, "Let's test her." She was being breast-fed, and they told [my daughter] to stop eating dairy. So my daughter went on a dairy-free diet. But the baby continued to have lots and lots of stomach cramps.

When she was 6 months old, they went to an allergy clinic and were told that under one she was too young for the blood tests for allergies to be meaningful at all, but that they'd do a blood test anyway. And the allergies to a number of things showed up in the super-high zone.

She was allergic to salmon, nuts, eggs, and dairy. She's now three and a half and goes every six months to the clinic. And it got more complicated. Now it's sesame seeds, tree nuts, and peanuts as well as dairy and eggs and most fish.

Fortunately she's never choked and turned blue. But her reaction to surface contact is high. When she was at a wedding with her parents and someone spilled a cup of coffee with milk in it on her leg, she got hives all over her body because of the teaspoon of milk in the coffee. She got hives from playgroup where some of the babies were drinking milk out of a bottle. Maybe it got on their hands [and then they] touched hers, or [it was on] a common surface.

She has to be watched all the time.

(MARY, 67)

Food allergies are caused by an inappropriate response of the immune system to an otherwise harmless substance. The trigger of this response appears to involve a combination of genetic and environmental factors. It is also unclear why food allergies are being diagnosed at such an increased rate. The increased use of antibiotics and their effect on the makeup of the microbiome has been implicated. Others blame processed foods and/or the emphasis on "clean" living—the hygiene hypothesis. This last theory is based on the premise that exposure is not a bad thing and allows the immune system to develop a more complete tolerance to foreign proteins. (See chapter 3, "The Hygiene Hypothesis.")

Some people believe that a mother's eating habits during pregnancy also play a role but this has not been scientifically proven. A mother's antibodies are protective and can cross the placenta during pregnancy and even during breast-feeding. But their direct effect as a protective mechanism in the gut is being questioned. For example, it was believed that starting gluten exposure in an infant during breast-feeding was protective against celiac disease, but this was disproved in a recent large study.

How Food Allergies Are Diagnosed

Currently, diagnosis relies on the presence of IgE antibodies in the blood. Yet the detection of specific IgE antibodies in blood tests and skin-prick tests are neither completely accurate nor reliable indicators of allergy. Therefore a careful medical history, and for some a food challenge, in addition to lab tests is recommended for diagnosis. Most panels for food allergies test for the "Big 8" major allergens. Elimination diets that take all potential allergens out of the diet for six weeks and then reintroduce them, one by one, are also utilized.

Treating Food Allergies

The management of food allergies requires the avoidance of the food(s) causing the reaction, and an appropriate and rapid response to the allergic reaction. Many patients carry an EpiPen (injected epinephrine to treat anaphylaxis) and/or Benadryl tablets in case of an unexpected exposure.

Studies and trials are under way to increase tolerance to various food allergens utilizing oral immunotherapy. Vaccines, Chinese herbal medicines, and anti-IgE antibodies are also being studied. The effectiveness of these therapies varies among different food antigens, and their long-term safety is also unclear. Other treatments involving sublingual (under the tongue) and epicutaneous (delivered through the skin) immunotherapy are being studied. At this point, their benefits and safety have not been fully demonstrated.

Many childhood food allergies resolve with age, and some people develop food allergies as adults.

Summary

- Food allergies are common and can be fatal. They cause an immediate immune reaction to the offending allergen. They are IgE mediated and different from the IgA- and IgG-mediated reactions associated with celiac disease and gluten sensitivity.

- The "hygiene hypothesis," which is based on the premise that early exposure to germs, infections, and foods is not necessarily a bad thing, has developed as one intriguing reason behind the increase in allergies. It is thought that exposure enables the immune system to develop tolerance and helps prevent allergies and some autoimmune diseases.

- Another intriguing hypothesis connects the increased use of antibiotics, especially in children, to disruptions or imbalances in the microbiome (*dysbiosis*) that in turn may account for some of the increase in childhood allergies.

- Allergies are another piece of the emerging food-gut-microbiome picture.

25

Fibromyalgia and Chronic Fatigue Syndrome

The greatest evil is physical pain.
—ST. AUGUSTINE

My auto accident at sixteen was the initial onset of my extreme fatigue and fogginess. But throughout college, the fatigue got worse and I started getting different joint and soft tissue pain. But because I was an active person, I would just brush it off.

When I was in my twenties, [my husband and I] lived in Germany, and when I was in elevations—like in the mountains—I would have trouble walking. And having babies was very difficult—my pregnancies were all very hard. I had a lot of pain in my shoulders and lower back.

In my thirties, I started thinking, *There has to be more to this,* and I started looking for answers. I started swimming and having massages, and started to try sensible eating, but nobody really knew why I was still so tired and had all these pains. The fatigue never dissipated.

(ANN, 71)

Fibromyalgia and chronic fatigue syndrome (also referred to as myalgic encephalomyelitis) are two diseases that have resisted neat medical categories—neurologic, rheumatic, and psychological—but cause fatigue and pain that can disrupt a life. Many people suffering with them believe that various exclusion diets are helpful, but others find them of little or no help. This has not kept alternative medicine practitioners from prescribing supplements and various diets—including a gluten-free diet—to treat the pain and fatigue people report.

Fibromyalgia

Fibromyalgia has been described as a problem with "volume control." The word *fibromyalgia* comes from the Latin *fibro* ("fibrous tissue") and the Greek *myo* (muscle) and *algia* (pain). It is characterized by chronic pain throughout the body, joint stiffness, and/or extremely tender musculoskeletal "trigger" points. The symptoms also include fatigue, problems sleeping, cognitive dysfunction, and mood and memory issues.

What Causes Fibromyalgia?

The causes of fibromyalgia are unknown, but there are probably a number of factors involved. The perceived pain appears to be related to biological, psychological, and sociological factors, as well as alterations or inflammation in the nervous system and its transmitters. Like Ann, many people associate the onset of fibromyalgia with a physically or emotionally stressful or traumatic event, repetitive injuries, or an illness. For others, fibromyalgia seems to occur spontaneously.

Many researchers are examining other causes, including problems with how the central nervous system processes pain. This syncs with the belief that fibromyalgia may be a condition of "central nervous system hypersensitivity" resulting in an amplified response to pain and stimuli. The problem has been in identifying the trigger of this sensitivity.

Researchers studying idiopathic (of unknown origin) pain disorders such as IBS and fibromyalgia believe that psychological distress and strong emotions play an important role in promoting the symptoms.

Some scientists speculate that there may be a genetic link in the way people process painful stimuli. Several genes that occur more commonly in fibromyalgia patients have already been identified.

How Is Fibromyalgia Diagnosed?

Since pain and fatigue are symptoms that occur in many other conditions, all of these must be ruled out before a diagnosis of fibromyalgia can be reached. Patients typically visit a number of doctors before getting a diagnosis, since standard laboratory tests often fail to reveal a physiological reason for the pain. Because there is no generally accepted, objective test for fibromyalgia, some doctors unfortunately may conclude that a patient's pain is not real, or they may tell the patient that little can be done.

A diagnosis can be made based on criteria established by the American College of Rheumatology that includes:

- tenderness in more than 19 pain locations
- six self-reported symptoms including difficulty sleeping, fatigue, poor cognition, headache, depression, and abdominal pain
- a history of widespread pain lasting more than three months

It is important that other conditions whose symptoms mimic fibromyalgia be ruled out. These include celiac disease, Lyme disease, arthritis, chronic fatigue syndrome, hypothyroidism, irritable bowel syndrome, lupus, and polymyalgia rheumatica. Some scientists have proposed that a percentage of patients with fibromyalgia suffer from underlying gluten sensitivity. Many symptoms of the two conditions are similar.

Conversely, some patients are given a diagnosis of fibromyalgia without proper lab testing, and are later found to have a treatable condition such as celiac disease.

How Is Fibromyalgia Treated?

I went to doctors who offered drugs and operations. I became addicted to painkillers and Valium because that's all they had to offer me. Fortunately, I had my own business—I had a job and a family—so I had a reason to keep going . . . I kept pursuing different avenues.

But I never got the connections to what I was eating until much, much later. In addition to the pain and fatigue, I've had irritable bowel syndrome for the past 15 years. Certain foods would make everything spasm. I constantly read and researched and tried things because my doctors didn't have answers.

In my 50s I started seeing some of the patterns but didn't know what to do with all the information. I was working hard on my diet but was given a lot of different ones. I knew that yeast was a problem in my body, and then I removed sugar and it seemed to be better. The white flour came later. I'm off dairy, gluten, sugar.

I found that diet and rest and exercise were the three things that kept me feeling better. I find that I'm in the water just about every day doing water aerobics classes, so I'm using the buoyancy of the water to help me. Going to a gym with a regular trainer and yoga got way too painful for me.

For years I've also done massage therapy and gone to support groups. Two other things are very helpful: aromatherapy and essential oils. I use those for pain instead of pills. I've never taken aspirin or anything for pain since the time I was addicted to pain pills.

(ANN, 71)

Fibromyalgia treatment is based on symptom control, which varies since every patient has a different level of physical and/or psychosocial distress. Many patients use a multifaceted approach that includes health care professionals, physical therapy, fitness training, cognitive behavioral therapy, acupuncture, and relaxation training. Most important, the patient must play an active role. The aim is the improvement of quality of life.

The FDA has approved several medications for the treatment of fibromyalgia but a recent study recommended that treatment for fibromyalgia using pharmaceuticals start "slow and low."

Doctors also treat fibromyalgia with a variety of other medications developed and approved for other purposes. Analgesics such as NSAIDs have been used to ease pain but are not effective at eradicating it. Antidepressants are also used to modulate pain.

Various dietary interventions have been investigated in fibromyalgia, and the findings were variable, ranging from negative to significantly effective.

> Today I don't think of myself as sick—and I think that also has had a tremendous effect. Am I symptom free? No, but I get in the pool or take a nap or ride my bike (I got a tricycle) or meditate—I know how to make myself feel better. The water has been a godsend. Exercise of the right kind is terribly important.
>
> I think if I didn't have the inner strength and positive outlook through the years, I would have been a shut-in.
>
> (ANN, 71)

Chronic Fatigue Syndrome

Chronic fatigue syndrome (CFS) is a condition that causes marked long-term tiredness (fatigue), headaches, difficulty concentrating, sleep disturbances, and other symptoms that are not caused by any other known medical condition. The core symptoms are a sustained depletion of energy after minimal activity and profound ongoing fatigue.

Many experts and patients prefer the term *myalgic encephalomyelitis*

(ME), meaning "brain and spinal cord inflammation with muscle pain," or ME/CFS, because it underscores a physical basis for the condition. Although some research has suggested that inflammation of the central nervous system is involved, its role is not proven, and muscle pain is not as prominent as other features.

What Causes CFS?

Several factors have been suggested in the development of CFS, including genetic, viral, immunological, neuroendocrine, and psychological. While the exact causes of CFS are unknown, it appears to be triggered by a variety of factors in people who have an underlying predisposition. Some suggest that it may be part of a double hit—after a viral infection that initiates an inflammatory response—but there is little scientific evidence to support this theory.

A recent study showed that there are changing levels of cytokines (molecules that stimulate or inhibit immune cells) in the blood samples of people with ME/CFS, indicating some kind of inflammatory and/or disease process at work. These biomarkers also indicate that people are not imagining or "making up" their symptoms. The role of these markers in the initiation or aggravation of the syndrome is under study.

How Is CFS Diagnosed?

There are currently no diagnostic lab tests or criteria that can confirm the diagnosis. It is made based on a pattern of symptoms and, more important, by excluding other conditions and diseases with similar symptoms.

The diagnosis is made after symptoms have persisted for at least three to four months and other conditions have been ruled out.

How Is CFS Treated?

Like fibromyalgia, CFS is treated by symptom control. This may include drugs, dietary changes, exercise routines, and cognitive therapy under professional guidance and medical supervision. Severe symptoms may require the support of a specialist in the condition.

Patients often feel that dietary manipulation can help to ease the fatigue—removing sugar, gluten, dairy, and/or other foods. Whether this is because of an underlying sensitivity to specific foods is unclear.

Before removing gluten from your diet, it is important to test first to make sure that you do not have celiac disease. After a period on a gluten-free diet, it may be impossible to diagnose this underlying condition without a gluten challenge, which requires adding gluten back to your diet.

Some patients with ME/CFS have low L-carnitine levels (see "Carnitine Supplements" in chapter 17, "Celiac Disease") and may benefit from supplements to improve their fatigue.

Are Fibromyalgia, Chronic Fatigue Syndrome, and Nonceliac Gluten Sensitivity Related?

Fatigue, brain fog, and joint and muscle pain are common symptoms in people who diagnose themselves as gluten sensitive. It is very possible that we are going to find gluten sensitivity in certain people with chronic fatigue syndrome and fibromyalgia.

We are currently analyzing blood samples to determine if they contain antibodies to gluten (antigliadin antibodies). As discussed before, the meaning of these antibodies is unclear—they do not indicate celiac disease but do indicate some type of immune response to dietary gluten. A gluten-free diet may help these specific patients. The antibodies may also be part of an inflammatory reaction that may yield a biomarker for these conditions.

Since the symptoms mimic those of celiac disease, it is possible that some people with fibromyalgia and chronic fatigue syndrome have an immune response to gluten that is similar to those with various neurological and psychiatric syndromes seen in celiac disease. This raises many interesting questions regarding the role of gluten in various neuromuscular conditions.

Summary

- Fibromyalgia and chronic fatigue syndrome are painful, stressful, and often debilitating conditions that are difficult to diagnose and treat. Most treatments aim to turn down the volume of the pain and eliminate or ease the level of fatigue.

- Because of the lack of clear-cut medical guidelines and specific biomarkers in patients with these conditions, many medical doctors dismiss the symptoms or prescribe painkillers. Unable to get direction from their doctors and seeking a diagnosis, patients are vulnerable to practitioners who subject them to expensive tests not covered by insurance and arduous therapies for the wrong condition. Others recommend expensive supplements and restricted diets. The diets appear to help some—if only to feel temporarily better—but the cost of most of the supplements is high and the benefits are low. Some supplements are dangerous and cause more harm than good.

- If taking control of your diet initiates a greater involvement in taking control of your body and the condition itself, the psychological benefit outweighs the effect of the food elimination.

PART V

The Brain-Gut-Gluten Connection

The human brain has 100 billion neurons, each neuron connected to 10 thousand other neurons. Sitting on your shoulders is the most complicated object in the known universe.
—MICHIO KAKU

If the body be feeble, the mind will not be strong.
—THOMAS JEFFERSON

Recent books and articles have called gluten the "silent killer" of the brain, claiming that whole grains cause dementia, autism, headaches, depression, anxiety, ADHD, and more. The scientific truth is that *reading and believing* this about grains probably fogs more brain cells than eating them will.

Our brains do exist in intimate interaction with our gut, where our "second brain" and our microbiome reside. But the direction of this interaction and who is in charge of which function is unclear. In fact, gut-microbiome-brain interactions offer insights into brain function in both health and disease. Whether this will have direct therapeutic results or prove to be only a small piece in a much larger brain-gut puzzle remains to be revealed. There are many more questions than scientific answers for this particular puzzle.

Brain study is in its infancy—we are still "orienteering." This is an activity where people are given a map and a compass, and navigate from point to point in unfamiliar territory to find something. Similarly, medical researchers are navigating a diverse and usually unfamiliar terrain to determine how, why, and if foods are the culprit in a number of psychiatric and neurological conditions.

Despite the many books and articles trumpeting clear connections, it is currently way too early to make scientific claims for specific or functional links between brain function, our microbiota, and gluten. What we do know is that intriguing pathways have been identified and that researchers are actively exploring them.

26

Autism Spectrum Disorders and ADHD

If we want to solve a problem that we have never solved before, we must leave the door to the unknown ajar.
—RICHARD P. FEYNMAN

According to various studies, gluten-free and/or casein-free diets are used by between 15 and 38 percent of parents for children on the autism spectrum. While the diets are increasingly popular, the theories and findings that are portrayed in the popular press, on websites, and in books appear to be more firmly established than the science behind them.

> When you first get a diagnosis, what you want is a way out, you want hope, you want treatment. So you're drawn to the promise of something.
>
> (DONNA, 42)

Parents are looking for treatments to do something, and specific foods are an appealing answer. There is a misconception that gluten is exacerbating or causing the symptoms of autism. So some parents immediately put their children on a gluten-free and/or casein-free diet in hopes that it will "cure" them.

Autism Spectrum Disorder

Autism spectrum disorder (ASD) is a disorder of neural development. It is characterized by impaired social communication and restrictive and repetitive behaviors. Many children have language and physical difficulties as well.*

There is no one clear cause of ASD, but contributing risk factors include:

- genes—ASD runs in families. If one sibling is diagnosed, a second sibling will have a 15 to 20 percent chance of developing the condition.
- sex—Males are four times more likely to have ASD.
- other environmental and/or biological factors

Ultimately, the odds are low that specific environmental insults such as paternal age or maternal infection that have been the focus of recent studies will influence the outcome. Other risk factors for autism are being studied. For example, researchers are looking at the effect of alterations in a young child's microbiome to see the impact on the development of autism. (See page 248, "ASD and the Microbiome.")

Symptoms of ASD emerge during early childhood and are typically diagnosed between 2 and 4 years of age. Diagnosis is done by a clinician based on behavioral observation and reports from parents.

There are currently no biomarkers or medical tests to diagnose ASD. Some genes have been implicated in the development of the disorder, but genes alone do not determine the onset of the condition.

Typical treatments include behavioral, speech, and physical therapies.

---

* The classification of Asperger's syndrome is no longer included in the latest revision of the *Diagnostic and Statistical Manual of Mental Disorders (DSM-V)*, which is used by professionals as the standard criteria by which to diagnose mental disorders. Children with these symptoms are considered to have high-functioning ASD.

There are currently no pharmaceutical treatments but research is being conducted on possible targets and drugs.

((Mommy, My Tummy Hurts))

[Our son] has chronic constipation and takes Miralax on a daily basis—it keeps things under control and his behavior under control as well.

Before we figured out what to use, he went for two to three days or more without a movement. You could see that he was upset—he wants to do it, and when he fails he gets upset and does more self-stimulation. You can't get his attention—he's in a zone. He won't engage in normal activities if he's very constipated.

(MARTY, 45)

Gastrointestinal complaints and conditions are among the most common medical issues associated with ASD. Diarrhea, constipation, and GERD are often reported. This may be a direct effect of certain behaviors ("holding it in" may result in constipation), or the GI complaint may affect their behavior as well as their physical well-being.

Many nonverbal children who cannot simply say that their tummies hurt express distress in other ways. A child in pain may withdraw or engage in self-injurious behavior (i.e., bite him- or herself) or have a tantrum in order to get attention so that someone will come to help. This does not mean that all children who display disruptive behaviors are masking GI symptoms; and GI issues are not seen as a singular problem in ASD—a subset of neurotypical children also have GI issues—but GI symptoms may be an extra barrier to ameliorate symptoms and affect treatment.

One recent study by Pat Levitt, Ph.D., a neuroscientist and professor at USC, showed that parents were aware of the existence but not necessarily the nature of a GI disorder in their child. And that a large portion of children in the study with GI disorders and ASD lacked "expressive language" and showed increased social impairment compared to those children with ASD who did not have GI issues. The study noted that this "novel finding . . . warrants further study." It was unclear whether the GI medical issues affected the child's ability to respond to treatment or whether the lack of expressive language itself contributed to constipation by "limiting appropriate toileting behavior."

Individuals with GI issues and ASD need to be diagnosed and treated by a gastroenterologist in order to isolate and properly treat their symptoms.

Visiting the Gastroenterologist

Taking a child with ASD to the doctor can pose a challenge. Many children are sensitive to new environments, and the doctor's office has a variety of unknowns including smells, sounds, and unfamiliar people. Preparing a child with ASD for some of the unknowns—what the situation will look like and what will happen—can help to reduce anxiety and agitation.

Autism Speaks, a nonprofit organization dedicated to research and information for the ASD community, has a comprehensive Parent's Guide to medical appointments and blood work. Links can be found in Appendix B, "Resources."

Why a Gluten-Free and/or Casein-Free Diet?

The role of gluten in the development, progress, and treatment of ASD is complex and under intense scrutiny in different settings. It is possible that the presence of IgG antigliadin antibodies may indicate a subset of children who may benefit from a gluten-free diet. (See chapter 6, "What Do Antibodies Tell Us?")

Studies have shown that there are increased food antibodies (IgG antigliadin antibodies and anticasein antibodies) in a subset of children with autism who have GI symptoms. These are nonceliac antibodies. While this suggests a gut-brain interaction, we do not know the direction of this interaction (i.e., is the brain affecting gut permeability or vice versa?). The presence of antibodies has to be shown to have a direct effect on brain function or dysfunction if it is to have scientific significance as a causative factor. Nevertheless, this immune response may help to identify novel biomarkers of ASD and offer new insights into the disease mechanisms for some of those with ASD.

A study of children with attention deficit hyperactivity disorder (ADHD) also showed that a subset had IgG antigliadin antibodies, but their significance is similarly unknown. Some experts feel that tests for antigliadin antibodies and the specific celiac antibodies should be part of the diagnostic process for these children to rule out celiac disease and to determine a possible sensitivity to gluten. The causes of ADHD are not known, but genes and environmental factors (maternal smoking and alcohol use, lead exposure, brain trauma) may contribute to symptoms. The roles of sugar and food additives have been studied with mixed scientific results. Some parents report that a sugar-free, gluten-free diet has improved hyperactive behaviors. Scientific studies have not objectively shown that elimination diets are effective in treating the symptoms of ADHD. It is fairly common that children with ASD may have symptoms of ADHD.

Several rationales are suggested to explain the presence of antibodies to gluten and casein in some people with ASD.

- The "leaky gut" theory suggests that impaired intestinal permeability allows harmful peptides, including gluten and casein, to diffuse into the body, where they create an immune response in the form of antibodies. (See chapter 16, "Intestinal Permeability.")
- Gluten may trigger an inflammatory response in the gut of some children, which may react with the central nervous system.
- A study found a significantly higher IgG antibody response to casein and gluten in patients with ASD in comparison to neurotypical

individuals, perhaps an indication of systemic inflammation that could include the gut.

- It is possible that altered intestinal permeability is a secondary effect that results from disturbed brain function (see the discussion on cerebral palsy in chapter 27, "Schizophrenia"), neither causing nor contributing to the brain dysfunction.

The exact significance of the presence of IgG antigliadin antibodies in this subset of people with ASD is unclear. Nevertheless, these individuals do appear to have more GI symptoms.

Most of the research studies following the effectiveness of gluten-free and/or casein-free diets in ASD have been shown to be too small to be statistically valid and/or flawed. Many rely on the reports of a parent or caregiver and may be influenced by the caregiver's desire for a positive outcome.

For the 1 percent of children with ASD who also have celiac disease, a gluten-free diet may have a dramatic effect on outcome. For those with nonspecific IgG antibodies to gluten, it may be helpful in alleviating symptoms, though this has not been demonstrated. For many others, isolating other causes for GI symptoms may be the most helpful way to resolve them.

Unfortunately, parents often receive conflicting advice about dietary interventions. While food and the GI tract are very clear issues for many individuals with autism, the science underlying the complex brain-gut puzzle is not.

When the twins got their diagnosis, it was a weeklong assessment that involved seeing a lot of specialists of different disciplines. And one of them was a psychiatrist. He was actually one of the most helpful, but at the end he wanted us to cut the boys off dairy completely for three months—he said it was just to see if it had an effect on their behavior. And he gave us forms to fill out for every day describing their behavior.

This was incredibly daunting, to say the least, having just received the autism diagnosis. And when we discussed this with the developmental pediatrician who was in essence the lead of the whole process, she actually rolled her eyes, and she said, "You're going through enough—no reason you have to do that. They need their dairy."

So, literally from the day of the diagnosis, we had two doctors telling us opposite things. To me the most daunting thing was that having gotten the diagnosis, there was no clear guidance as to what was real and what was not real.

Our disposition from the beginning, because of our experience with the two specialists, was to doubt dietary interventions.

(MARTY, 45)

Pitfalls of a Gluten-free Diet for People with ASD

There are many feeding issues in children with ASD. They are more "picky" eaters than those in the general population, perhaps a manifestation of restricted and repetitive behaviors that are a hallmark of the disorder. A gluten-free diet is often low in fiber and essential nutrients, and this may only compound the problem. Recent studies on the presence of heavy metals in people on a gluten-free diet raise possible neurological complications that need to be studied further. (See chapter 4, "Pitfalls and Perils of a Gluten-Free Diet.")

[My son's] teachers sometimes use food rewards when something requires a very high motivation, like during the first stages of toilet training. Now they use an activity they like. In most schools I had to send them the edible rewards. So you have that control over it.

(DONNA, 42)

A restrictive diet is also difficult to enforce—children with ASD often see many different therapists and clinicians in the course of a typical school day (speech, art, movement therapy). Often, each group uses food as a reward to enforce desired behaviors. If that reward is a cookie or cracker with gluten, it may trump efforts to keep to a gluten-free diet. Thus parents may be seeing results that relate more to therapy than to diet.

> Feeding my son is incredibly hard work.
>
> (SALLY, 36)

For some children with ASD, feeding and/or eating takes on a life of its own. A preference for specific foods—yellow or red, mushy or crunchy, spicy or bland—and sensory sensitivity can limit diets and create behavioral issues as well as malnutrition.

A gluten-free diet is a popular consideration for this population, but has not been demonstrated to alter the disorder state. It may also be extremely difficult to enforce, adding additional stress to family meals.

ASD and the Microbiome

It has been hypothesized that changes in the gut microbiome play a role in the development of ASD. These studies are further complicated by the fact that individuals with autism frequently receive medication with antibiotics, are often on special diets, are highly dietary selective, and/or have repetitive dietary behaviors, all of which may alter their microbiota. Thus, it is difficult to establish whether the changes are causative or simply a consequence of the disease or its treatment.

Since it is difficult to study the human gut at a molecular level, some researchers have studied the influence of the microbiota on brain development and function in ASD on specially bred mice. These studies have established a link between the microbiota and autism-like behaviors, but not the underlying mechanisms. That is, it is not clear whether alterations in the gut microbiota are causing autism symptoms.

Some studies indicate that the serotonin system is involved in the development of GI symptoms in ASD. (See "The Molecular Busybody" in chapter 10, "The 'Second Brain'.") These studies involve mice with a genetic mutation from humans with ASD affecting GI and serotonin function. The mouse does not have autism but genetic permutations and features that are similar to humans with ASD. This research has provided information about the relationships between diet and the microbiome in a specific subset of people with ASD. While mice are not, as a recent article noted, "little humans with tails," they open a window into the relationship between diet, the microbiome, and GI complaints.

What Does It All Mean?

Although the links are currently unclear, it is possible that breakthrough autism treatments may start in the GI tract. Researchers are studying whether GI symptoms are a manifestation of the neurodevelopmental disorder that could be a clue to its physical and biochemical development. An article in *Autism Speaks* notes, "Studies that improve our understanding of these brain-gut connections are laying a pathway to innovations in treatment."

It is increasingly frustrating for the parents and caretakers of individuals with ASD to continually hear "it's unclear" and "we don't know what will work or what this means." What is clear is the importance of correctly testing for, diagnosing, and treating GI disorders in this population. *Anyone* in pain or suffering from GI distress will have difficulty focusing on mental tasks. This can have distinct repercussions on the many interventions used to treat ASD.

Summary

- The use of gluten-free and/or casein-free diets in people with ASD is controversial. Scientific studies have not proven objective changes in behaviors for children on these diets.

- Parents should be aware of the serious pitfalls of a gluten-free diet before implementing one for their child. They are adding nutritional as well as food choice limitations to a population already burdened by restrictions.

- The presence of antibodies to gluten in a subset of children with ASD is an intriguing finding and may point to a group of people who might benefit from a gluten-free diet. But these antibodies must be studied further to determine when they develop and how this relates to the child's development. We must be careful not to confuse association with cause.

- Gastrointestinal dysfunction may provide a window to better understand both autism and the brain in autism. It is a bidirectional avenue that may hold answers even in those without GI disorders. Potentially it could mean that a drug targeting the intestines might help neuropsychiatric conditions.

27

Schizophrenia—Revisiting "Bread Madness"

Science is like a love affair with nature; an elusive,
tantalizing mistress. It has all the turbulence, twists and
turns of romantic love, but that's part of the game.
—VILAYANUR S. RAMACHANDRAN

The evidence for a connection between disturbances in the GI tract and psychiatric illness has been accumulating for many years. Our growing understanding of how the brain, the microbiome, and the enteric nervous system—the "second brain" in the gut—interact has uncovered intriguing associations between what we ingest and behavior. But as we must consistently note in this section focusing on the brain, there is a big difference between association and cause.

Bread Madness

The association of bread with madness dates back to the Middle Ages, when rye was susceptible to ergot, a fungus containing chemicals that resemble LSD. When eaten, it caused convulsions, pain, and a type of "madness" called St. Anthony's Fire, or ergot poisoning. The symptoms became associated with "bewitching" and may have accounted for some of the accusations behind the Salem Witch Trials. The "madness" symptoms were then attached to schizophrenia. In the 1920s, the "intestinal intoxication" theory of schizophrenia was popular. Papers in the 1960s referred to schizophrenia as "bread madness."

This lingering belief has been replaced—at least in the scientific community—with an understanding that while the specific causes of schizophrenia are unknown, contributing factors appear to include a genetic predisposition interacting with complex environmental and neurotransmitter disturbances. But intriguing connections to gluten remain.

They exist in the similarity of genes for schizophrenia and certain genes found in other autoimmune disorders such as celiac disease. An infectious "insult"—exposure to the parasite *Toxoplasma gondii*—is a known risk factor for the development of schizophrenia, presumably through a direct effect of the parasite on brain and behavior. This may also be part of a "double hit" where an infection with toxoplasmosis combined with an immune response to gluten in susceptible individuals can result in schizophrenia. (Also see chapter 14, "The Double Hit Theory.") Dr. Robert Yolken, an investigator from Johns Hopkins University, has provided evidence supporting this theory.

Some researchers hypothesize that an alteration of gut permeability may be the initial step causing both schizophrenia and celiac disease, sharing similar pathways of altered gut permeability. In this scenario, the gut of genetically susceptible people may lose its capacity to block toxins and psychosis-causing substances may enter the body, thus causing the development of various psychiatric conditions.

The microbiome may also play a part, since manipulation of the microbiota in germ-free animals has created behavioral as well as biochemical and molecular changes.

The Presence of Anti-gliadin Antibodies—
The Horse or the Cart?

Studies show that some patients with schizophrenia have *IgG antigliadin antibodies*. These antibodies are also associated with neurologic and psychiatric manifestation (ataxia, peripheral neuropathies, brain fog) but without the GI symptoms seen in celiac disease. (See "What Do Antibodies to Gluten Really Mean?" in chapter 6, "Testing.")

It has been proposed that the IgG antigliadin antibodies seen in these patients reflect an increased sensitivity or immunological response to gliadin. This does not appear to affect the GI tract, but it has been suggested that the antibodies cross-react with parts of the central nervous system or specific proteins in the brain.

While it is hoped that a resolution of antibodies would improve symptoms in schizophrenia, studies with gluten-free diets have had mixed results. None of these studies, however, have focused on those most likely to respond—those with antigliadin antibodies. It is clear that the gut-brain interaction goes both ways. What is not clear is whether gluten sensitivity is the result of, or contributes to, the development or progression of this disease.

The effect of these antibodies on function cannot be proven as yet. They may very well be a good measure of the wrong thing.

Cerebral Palsy

Cerebral palsy (CP) results from "insults" to different areas of the developing nervous system and causes a varying severity of symptoms. The management of these symptoms is the goal of treatment, and children with severe spasticity often suffer from problems with swallowing, reflux, and delayed stomach emptying. This can lead to malnutrition.

An increased level of IgG antibodies to gliadin as well as other food components has also been found in some patients with cerebral palsy. The clinical implications of their presence in this condition are unclear. They do, however, indicate that the gut-brain interaction is bidirectional—CP is primarily a brain problem, yet there are increased food antibodies.

In one interesting study, positive IgG antigliadin antibodies to gliadin were found in children with CP who had lower weight, height, and BMI compared to healthy children. A number of possible reasons were suggested, focusing on an effect on the gut that was not recognized, an inflammation of the gut mucosa, or intestinal permeability leading to an immune response in the body.

While some parents put children with cerebral palsy on a gluten-free and/or casein-free diet, the pitfalls of the diet should be taken into account in children whose nutritional status may be at risk. (See chapter 4, "Pitfalls and Perils of a Gluten-Free Diet.") The benefits of the diet at this point appear to be very controversial and may be harmful for children already suffering from malnutrition.

Summary

Various neuropsychological conditions highlight the complex brain-gut connection. Clearly more research is needed to determine if IgG antigliadin antibodies and other food antibodies are a marker of blood-brain barrier disruption and contribute to brain dysfunction. If so, it would provide an impetus for examining the effect of a gluten-free diet in a subset of patients who have antibodies to gluten.

This is an exciting field of research that may help provide evidence that links disrupted pathways outside of the brain to the development of certain brain disorders.

28

Brain Fog—Neurology
or Meteorology?

After only one month on a [gluten-free] diet, I felt as if a veil had
been lifted from my brain.

(ROZ, 58)

"Brain fog" is one of the most common symptoms mentioned by people
with gluten-related disorders. It is not an acknowledged medical term but
a definition that originated with patients. It is described as mental confusion, a lack of clarity or focus, and forgetfulness.

The mechanisms causing these symptoms are unclear, but the same
symptoms can be caused by a number of factors including lack of sleep,
various neurological disorders, stress, early stages of dementia, diabetes
(fluctuating glucose levels can affect brain function), chemotherapy (aka
"chemo fog"), anesthesia, acute illnesses, and the side effects of various
medications.

While the various tests to measure cognition and depression contain
limitations, different instruments are used to measure attention, concentration, orientation, short- and long-term memory, praxis (the ability to
learn and retain new information), speed of processing, language, and

executive function. The results would indicate that brain fog is very real in a subset of patients with celiac disease.

Brain fog is also considered a classic aspect of chronic fatigue syndrome and fibromyalgia, and is often accompanied by disorientation and difficulty in finding words.

In an intriguing new study, Peter Gibson, M.D., of Monash University in Australia looked at the cognitive function of people newly diagnosed with celiac disease. He found that the cognitive performance of one group of patients on a strict gluten-free diet showed a definite improvement that paralleled the healing in their gut. He concluded that "suboptimal levels of cognition in untreated celiac disease may affect the performance of everyday tasks."

Before going on a gluten-free diet, the subjects had a level of impairment similar to people with a blood alcohol level equal to the upper legal limit for driving in Australia. It is also the equivalent of severe jet lag. This meant that someone with untreated celiac disease might be at risk for impaired performance at work or while driving. In fact, a Swedish study found that asymptomatic young adults in whom celiac disease was discovered by screening had fewer university degrees and managerial positions compared to subjects in an age-matched control group.

Using five different research instruments and questionnaires, Gibson's group assessed subtle cognitive impairment, the recall of words, fine motor movements, and the reconstruction of complex situations. The study showed that all were impaired and improved at six and twelve months on the diet. This correlated with improved blood tests and biopsy results. The results suggest that there is a real impairment of cognitive function related to disease activity. That said, the mechanisms underlying these symptoms are not clear, and the results could be different for different individuals. More studies are needed to replicate these findings.

What Causes Brain Fog?

There are a number of theories on the development of brain fog in gluten-related disorders.

Inflammation

Many cellular markers are released during inflammation that permeate organs and signal the brain to induce a "sickness response." This includes symptoms such as fatigue, depression, lack of motivation, and lack of mental clarity that often clears up along with the disease. Most people experience this crawl-into-bed response when sick with the flu. In conditions such as irritable bowel syndrome, chronic inflammation provokes a transition from this type of sickness response into depression and chronic pain.

Cytokines (molecules that signal the inflammatory response) are one such marker released in response to infections, illness, and stress. The brain has cytokine receptors, and these cells may bind to neurons and affect signaling. If levels of these cells persist in the body they may cause a disruption of perception.

Several studies offer insights into the complex relationship between inflammatory processes and neurological function. Studies show that antibodies to gluten do bind to nervous tissue in humans and animals. In celiac disease specifically, we know that antigliadin antibodies can bind to proteins in neurological tissue. While it is unclear whether binding interferes with the function of the tissue, studies suggest that it does.

It is also possible that inflammation in the gut disrupts the microbiota that in turn affects the gut-brain pathway.

Gluten

When someone has an immune response to gluten, there is an increase in inflammatory mediators (e.g., cytokines) that might interfere with the blood-brain barrier or disrupt various hormones and enzymes. These disruptions may cause depression, cognitive impairment, or brain fog in some individuals.

Nutrient Deficiencies

There is a fair amount of evidence showing that vitamin deficiencies affect the nervous system. Patients with untreated celiac disease or other intestinal malabsorption conditions may have vitamin and mineral deficiencies affecting cognitive function and/or causing neurological deficits.

Gut Microbiota

The gut-brain-microbiome axis appears to plays a role in influencing brain development, mood, and behavior. In a similar vein, an unhealthy diet has recently been highlighted as a risk factor for depression.

Our gut microbiota interacts bi-directionally with environmental factors such as diet and stress, and this may eventually be a target for interventions to treat mental conditions. Studies of this are in very early stages, and no direct link to brain fog has been suggested.

Stress and Anxiety Due to Illness or Trauma

An illness itself may play a major role in initiating brain fog. Sickness can alter one's ability to function, and subtle cognitive functions like memory are more vulnerable to stress and anxiety.

Poor stress resilience and an exaggerated inflammatory response to environmental stress is characteristic of people who have undergone trauma in their early lives. This in turn may affect cognition and well-being. (For more, see chapter 29, "The Stress of Holding Back.")

Summary

- Any physical illness, whether acute or chronic, is usually accompanied by numerous psychological symptoms that may include fatigue, depression, an increased sensitivity to pain, and lack of motivation, appetite, and sociability. They are part of what is called a "sickness response," and most disappear with the disease.

- Brain fog may be a symptom or part of a sickness response in those with an immune or inflammatory response to gluten. The mechanisms underlying the condition are unclear, but the brain fog is real.

- If your illness is chronic, your sickness response may be as well. This might require pharmaceuticals to treat both the physical as well as psychological symptoms.

- Brain fog may be another piece of the conversation between the brain, the gut, and our microbiome. This puzzle is still missing many pieces, which scientists may be able to identify as targets for treatment in the future. At this point, a gluten-free diet clears the fog for some people with celiac disease, but should not be considered the dietary answer to treating brain fog in others.

29

The Stress of Holding Back

"Stressed" is "desserts" spelled backward.

—ANONYMOUS

College on a strict gluten-free diet is way harder than I expected. It's definitely not easy to balance schoolwork and also worry about food all the time! A lot of people here in California are on the gluten-free diet for the fad, which undermines the severity of celiac disease and cross-contamination and everything. It was a huge struggle. In college I've been more resentful of the disease than any time before. Social life is isolating, dealing with my own food. I often have to go back to my room to get something to eat, and that takes away that spontaneity that makes college so fun. I feel like I'm missing out. That's the most difficult [thing]. I constantly have to be vigilant. At home it's so nice to know that everything is safe—it's a lot more relaxing.

(ALEXIS, 20)

Is it a gluten-free diet—not the gluten—that is stressing your brain circuits and causing a literal brain drain?

Stress is defined as a physical, mental, or emotional factor that causes bodily or mental tension. There is good stress that keeps us alert and involved, and bad stress that takes a mental and physical toll. People who are always on alert when eating or living with a chronic illness have constant stress—a condition that loads the part of the brain responsible for executive function, tapping its resources and making it less effective. This eventually produces wear and tear on the entire body—referred to as "allostatic load" in the medical literature. This "load" is triggered by various chemicals and hormones released in response to stress, and can determine our patterns of emotional response and resiliency to events that can extend far beyond the dinner table.

The Evolutionary Perspective

Stress responses benefit animals in the wild and may have given our prehistoric ancestors a survival advantage in avoiding predators. Daniel Lieberman, an evolutionary biologist and professor at Harvard University, puts it most succinctly in noting that animals on the Serengeti do two things most of the day: "They eat and they worry."

These survival skills are not required when seeking food in the supermarket, but we now worry about gluten, fat, and carbohydrates rather than large predators—an evolutionary shift of focus that is affecting our brains and health in unexpected ways.

> I feel nervous whenever I'm on a date. Afraid he won't like me because I ask the waiter so many questions. Makes me a neurotic mess, I guess.
>
> (JOAN, 28)

While it is a highly subjective phenomenon that is difficult to measure, it is becoming increasingly clear that the stress of "holding back," of monitoring, measuring, and thinking about what we eat at every meal and in every social setting, has many silent and cumulative effects. Beyond the fight-or-flight response that characterizes acute stress, when food and eating become chronic concerns of everyday life, the stress can affect thought, mental performance, and the responses of numerous organs.

The Burden of Restrictive Dieting

Having a gluten-free home is expensive but manageable; the problem comes with outings, vacations and trips, and trying to go to
restaurants. And it seems like school is much more prepared and
willing to deal with peanut allergies and that sort of thing.

(RAY, 38)

For people with chronic illnesses such as celiac disease, IBS, IBD, type 1
diabetes, or a food allergy, stress comes in navigating a school cafeteria,
counting carbs, always reading labels, carrying an EpiPen, ordering in a
restaurant, and constantly being vigilant.

In a recent study, people with celiac disease perceived the treatment
burden of the diagnosis as a heavier one than end-stage renal failure (a
fatal condition in which the options are dialysis several times a week or
a kidney transplant). Many come to an entirely gluten-free event and
remark, "It was the first time I remember being so totally relaxed at a
party—I never worried about what I was putting in my mouth." Others
with IBS sometimes eat nothing at an event in fear of not reaching the
bathroom in time. Like individuals with a food allergy, they are on per-
petual alert, a stressful state of constant vigilance, where food is involved.

What Your Brain Gains and Loses
on a Diet of Chronic Stress

The brain is the main organ in the body that determines what we perceive as stressful and how we will react and adapt to it. It is also a target
of the stress, and this can have lasting effects on it. And there are enormous differences in how each individual responds. When stress becomes
a destructive element in someone's life, it is important to take steps to
address the consequences. Sometimes it is a silent pressure that only
shows its face after much damage is done.

Stress "loads" the prefrontal cortex, the part of our brain where executive function is centered. This function involves a number of abilities that affect your capacity to organize and manipulate different types of information and behaviors. It comes into play during decisions that involve planning, decision-making, abstract thinking, troubleshooting, initiating or inhibiting responses and/or temptations, and processing sensory information. It may actually play a role in the brain fog that many patients report. (See chapter 28, "Brain Fog.")

Stress can also affect impulse control because it elevates *glucocorticoid* levels, sometimes for extended periods of time. These steroid hormones regulate the body's need for energy. One of the glucocorticoids, cortisol, causes the body to crave food—many people say they "eat when stressed."

In teenagers, the prefrontal cortex is not yet fully developed—one reason many have poor impulse control in general. But impulse control is a complex phenomenon that is intertwined with other "reward" systems in the brain that are developing during adolescence. The combination of immature systems often results in poor choices within this age group that makes dietary and health constraints harder to follow.

There is also an increased sensitivity to pain that is often found in people suffering from chronic stress. This, however, is a two-way street. Not only is it possible that social distress may sensitize individuals to physical pain, enhanced pain may lead to greater perception of social distress. Researchers note that these two processes seem to be moving together and possibly influencing each other.

Adjusting to a Restricted Diet

A crust eaten in peace is better than a banquet partaken in anxiety.
—AESOP

There are many reasons a restricted diet is difficult, including the necessary change in habits, social and cultural constraints and stigma, and loss of control (of impulses and the ability to find "safe" food). Your adjustment will then depend on your personality and how you respond to the change. People who need to be in control can become extremely frustrated. While some psychologists recommend trying out "other ways to be in the world," this is not always easily achieved.

> What is it like to be the grandmother of a child with celiac disease?
> It's more a question of being the mother-in-law of the mother of the child with celiac disease.
>
> (LUCY, 65)

The timing and delivery of the diagnosis can affect the difficulty in dealing with the condition. When diagnosis comes during adolescence—a sensitive developmental period—the perceived negative effects are often more severe than during early childhood, when the condition is integrated into identity and habit more readily.

> My doctor said, "You have celiac disease. Go on a gluten-free diet, and I'll see you in six months." That's when we got really frustrated and really lost. My doctor sent me home without any guidance.
>
> (ALEXIS, 20)

Patients who receive excellent dietary counseling and guidance at the time of diagnosis are more accepting of the diagnosis and restrictions than those left to fend for themselves on the Internet.

Identity Threats

> It's interesting to watch my granddaughter develop her self-identity. Who she is is someone who cannot play with a child who has peanut butter on his hands. Who she is is someone who can never go into an ice cream store and eat regular ice cream. It's incorporated into her identity.
>
> (MARY, 67)

In a recent book on how stereotypes affect us, the social psychologist Claude M. Steele discusses how stereotype threats have a real effect on people.* And people on a very restricted diet are often marginalized and/ or made to feel an outsider to the food at parties, galas, business meals, school trips, and many restaurants. Some schools even refuse to take children with food allergies or intolerances on class trips where they cannot readily accommodate dietary restrictions that might cause a health issue.

Steele analyzed the effect when identity threats become chronic and are an ongoing experience in some area of one's life. His studies suggest that the long-term stress of dealing with threats to identity may undermine not only a person's happiness, but also contribute to health issues.

Fortunately, as Bruce McEwan, a neuroscientist and professor at Rockefeller University, emphasizes, "The good news is that interventions can prevent the negative effects of stress on the brain and body."

> I kept a gluten-free kitchen even when my daughter went off to college. This way she can relax completely and feel safe when she comes home.
>
> (AMY, 49)

Navigating Through the Stress of Holding Back

There are several steps you can take to improve your stress levels and your perception of stress.

1. Rewrite the Script

> You hear, "It's not fair, I don't get to eat what the other kids are eating."
> It actually is fair. It would be unfair for me to give my son what the

---

* Claude M. Steele, *Whistling Vivaldi* (New York: W.W. Norton & Co., 2010).

other kids are getting. What we can try to do is make things equivalent. So if they're getting a dessert, you might not get the same dessert, but you'll get the dessert that's good for you. That's fair.

We don't all get the same things out of life, but we can make them the equivalent.

(KEIRA, 43)

2. **Eat a Healthy Diet, Get Physical Activity, and Sleep**

Stress depletes the body—a balanced diet of fresh food, exercise, and sufficient hours of rest feed and restore it. Sleep deprivation also triggers hormones that stimulate hunger—studies have found that people who sleep less are more likely to be overweight.

3. **Get Social Support**

Eating is very personal, and many people feel it does not require outside intervention and interference. But people with chronic illnesses and allergies fare best when supported by medical professionals who understand the science behind their conditions. The support of family and friends can reduce the "solitary" burden and make social occasions easier to navigate. For example, celiac disease meet-ups have become increasingly popular in some cities and offer the exchange of restaurant and product suggestions that encourage compliance and comfort with the diagnosis, and grow social resilience through shared participation in a diagnosis and treatment.

4. **Try Different "Mind Practices"**

If compliance is difficult and causing medical issues, cognitive behavioral therapy (CBT) has been shown to be very effective in improving attitude and approach. Many patients with chronic fatigue syndrome, fibromyalgia, and IBS report that meditation and mindfulness also decrease painful symptoms and improve their quality of life.

You may need to set up a mental road map that differs from the patterns and routes you have been taking.

5. **Reward Yourself**

We all crave a treat or comfort food every so often and want to be rewarded for good behavior on a diet. People on a weight-loss diet are wisely counseled not to eat an entire piece of chocolate cake. When you *must* have one, take a few bites. This is where the advice to those on a gluten-free diet to find substitutes for their favorite foods—pizza, chocolate brownies, beer, mac and cheese, etc.—cannot be emphasized enough.

There is a difference between rewarding yourself with a safe food and cheating.

6. **Seek Out Medical Professionals to Help Manage Your Disease**

Keeping your disease and symptoms well managed will lower your stress levels. Far too many people who are prescribed a gluten-free diet are not advised to see a dietitian or feel they are expert and vigilant enough to teach their children and handle the diet on their own. Yet we have heard children admit to cheating on the diet when their parents were not present. Dropping off the diet is frequent at times of stress and transition—changing schools, entering college, a first or new job—and having direct access to a dietitian can make these transitions easier.

7. **Use Pharmaceutical Agents If Necessary**

There are a number of drugs used to control stress, including antidepressants, beta blockers, sleeping pills, and other agents for relief from inflammation and pain. All have strengths, limitations, and side effects that must be measured and balanced with your underlying condition as well as your level of stress.

Directing your energy toward the management and control of personal perception and behaviors can help the brain respond more flexibly to stress. As Professor McEwan states, "Motivation and decision making and perseverance are all functions of the brain!"

Holding back can create stress that eventually colors an individual's perception of food, family, friends, and lifestyle. Being aware of its impact on your brain and body can affect your long-term health and well-being.

PART VI

Navigating a Gluten-Free Life

Minds are like parachutes, they only function when open.
—THOMAS DEWAR

Things should be made as simple as possible—but not simpler.
—ALBERT EINSTEIN

The first five sections of this book put gluten and the gastrointestinal tract under the microscope. They examined the public perceptions—and misconceptions—about the grain, its role in different diseases and conditions, its effect on the GI tract and possibly the brain, and how a gluten-free diet and lifestyle can affect your stress level and resilience.

We also explored how everything we ingest affects the GI tract and why other foods, drugs, and toxins create the symptoms often attributed to gluten.

But the complete picture cannot be drawn without a closer inspection of the pharmaceutical drugs being developed to assist those on a gluten-free diet as well as the myths, hidden ingredients, food guidelines, and future directions for those trying to navigate a healthy and symptom-free life.

30

Nondietary Therapies— the Drug Pipeline

I can resist everything except temptation.
—OSCAR WILDE

It is difficult to follow a strict, lifelong diet of any type, but that is currently the only safe and effective treatment for those with celiac disease. Patients need and want a nondietary form of therapy for several reasons:

- Temptation, the desire to eat "some" gluten if symptoms are not severe, can make compliance a real problem, especially if there are no immediate symptoms when the gluten is ingested.
- Products, even those labeled "gluten-free," can be contaminated.
- A small percentage of patients do not respond to the diet, and an even greater number (estimated at 30 to 70 percent) do not heal completely.
- Patients with minimal symptoms prior to diagnosis may become more sensitive to gluten after a period on a gluten-free diet.

Various studies underscore the extent of these issues. One study of patients in the UK showed that 70 percent either intentionally and/or inadvertently ingested gluten. It is also hard to avoid gluten even in products marked "gluten-free." While there are only a few good studies, those that exist indicate that a few breakfast cereals marked as gluten-free contained amounts of gluten greater than the minimal amount allowed by law to carry that label. Gluten has also been found in various supplements, an unregulated industry where the "gluten-free" label currently is questionable.

A nondietary answer therefore holds tremendous appeal and has a long history in other GI conditions. Lactase pills, for example, have made having an ice cream cone or slice of pizza possible for those with lactose intolerance. And antacids are a staple in most households. They do not replace the need to avoid dairy or highly fatty foods for these individuals, but treat a dietary "mistake" or indiscretion. Severe IBD can be put into total symptomatic and histological remission.

All this has led to the development of some very promising and exciting alternative and/or complementary approaches to a gluten-free diet. Since more is known about the development of celiac disease than any other autoimmune disease, researchers have tracked the pathways through which the partially degraded and toxic fragment of gluten gets into the lining of the intestine and interacts with the immune system. It is these very pathways that are the target of various therapies.

While there is currently *no* product on the market that prevents, halts, or reduces the harmful effect of gluten on people with celiac disease, the following show the most promise at the moment. The potential therapies block, bind, or degrade the toxic components of gluten. **Except for the vaccine, they all currently work *in conjunction with* a gluten-free diet.**

> I'm the kind who, if you can take a pill for it, it's perfect. I'm ready when the pill is ready.
>
> (CHERRY, 35)

I'm leery of untested things in general. I'd be scared of trying the
new therapies until they've been on the market for a few years.

(NED, 52)

Helping Digest or Degrade Gluten

The gluten protein is not completely digested in the small intestine by
the proteases (enzymes that break down proteins) in our GI tract. But
a number of different proteases that do digest gluten exist in nature.
They are referred to often as glutenases and can come from various
sources.* They exist in some grains—including, ironically, barley—
and in bacteria and fungi. These sources are being harnessed to be
manufactured in commercial quantities with special qualities. They
can also be specifically engineered in the laboratory. They need to be
able to act fast and completely in the very acidic environment of the
stomach, while the stomach is mixing and dissolving ingested food,
and before it leaves to enter the small intestine. This is a very promising therapy.

Studies have demonstrated that some glutenase enzyme preparations can effectively digest gluten in the acidic environment of the
stomach. ALV003, manufactured in the U.S. from barley and bacteria,
and AN-PEP, manufactured in the Netherlands from fungi, appear
effective. However, placebo-controlled studies in patients with celiac
disease did not meet the planned primary end points of the studies. This emphasizes the difficulty in conducting placebo-controlled
studies in those with celiac disease. A promising, potent engineered
enzyme (Kuma030) is being studied by investigators at the University
of Washington.

---

* The suffix "–ase" is used to form the names of enzymes: lactase breaks down lactose, lipase breaks down lipids or fats, etc.

While other glutenases from various sources including mouth bacteria, stool bacteria, and probiotics have been detected, none have been commercially developed at this time.

It must be reiterated that there are currently many available OTC glutenases marketed as dietary supplements that have *not* been evaluated by the FDA and are *not* effective in degrading or digesting gluten in the stomach despite claims to the contrary. We recommend that patients with celiac disease specifically avoid using these products, as they could be harmful.

Inhibiting Intestinal Permeability

Larazotide Acetate

Another drug with FDA Fast Track designation, Larazotide, has a strategy based on keeping the toxic gliadin peptides from entering the intestinal lining, where they trigger the immune response. It essentially shuts the gate that lets the toxic peptides in.

Larazotide works on the "tight junctions" holding the cells together and may also be working on other components of the transport mechanisms between cells. Gluten is also transported *through* the epithelial cells, and Larazotide would not block this entry. (See chapter 16, "Intestinal Permeability.")

Phase II clinical trials have shown it to be effective and generally well tolerated in improving symptoms of celiac disease more than a gluten-free diet alone. To date, the studies have not included biopsies to assess mucosal injury, but they would be necessary for FDA approval and will be necessary end points in definitive trials.

Binding Gluten with Polymers to Safely Escort It from the GI Tract

BioLineRx Ltd.'s BL-7010

Distinct from therapies that degrade gluten, this approach uses polymers that act in the intestinal tract (the *lumen*). The polymers are being developed with the ability and properties necessary to target and bind gliadin and prevent digestion and absorption. It would then be "escorted" out of the GI tract and excreted in stool. Studies in experimental animals show that BL-7010 does do this. In the U.S., it has not yet progressed to clinical trials in humans, where it must be proven safe. There is concern that it can also block/bind with vitamins and minerals and prevent their absorption. This is an attractive form of therapy, since physicians prescribe a similar class of drugs to treat high cholesterol and diarrhea.

Vaccine to Induce Tolerance to Gluten

ImmusanT's Nexvax2

Nexvax2 is an injectable vaccine that is designed to induce immune tolerance to gluten. It is designed to work like an allergy shot—exposing the immune system in a controlled way. It is assumed that the vaccine will induce tolerance by acting on the T-cells, which serve as a go-between in the immune system, and create a protective T-cell response.

ImmusanT has identified three of the most potent peptides causing the immune reaction in people with HLA-DQ2–associated celiac disease. This accounts for approximately 90 percent of people with celiac disease. The vaccine will not work for patients who have the -DQ8 genes.

It has been tested in Phase I trials in Australia and shown to be safe and tolerable. It must now move to trials to test its effectiveness in protecting the intestine from gluten damage. This treatment would involve patients continuing to eat gluten and require regular injections—similar to someone receiving allergy shots.

If proven safe and effective, a vaccination strategy might be even more attractive than other novel treatments.

Other Potential Therapies

Blocking Tissue Transglutaminase

Tissue transglutaminase (tTG Inhibitor) is the enzyme that changes gluten into a toxic molecule for people with celiac disease. Therefore, inhibiting its action has been suggested as an effective therapeutic approach for celiac disease. Since tTG is also an essential enzyme used by the body for wound binding and other binding activities, it poses a high risk if the therapy blocks tTG in any other organ or interacts and/or disturbs other metabolic or biological pathways.

Studies on this approach are still preclinical (not conducted in humans).

Modifying Wheat

It has been proposed that modifying wheat strains to remove the peptides causing the immune reaction—without removing the baking quality of the wheat—might be an option for people with celiac disease seeking to replace gluten-containing bread.

There are many challenges in the process of the modification of gluten contents in the wheat varieties. Modifying the protein contents may lead to a loss of or decrease in baking characteristics; all the peptides in wheat that causes an immune reaction are still not known; the potential for contamination of genetically modified grains with the wild strains during cultivation, pollination, harvesting, and processing is possible; commercial wheat is cheap and any future genetically engineered wheat would increase in cost in an already price-inflated gluten-free market.

An alternative approach is to detoxify gluten by using bacteria-derived peptidases during food processing that would "digest" the wheat peptides. This is the process by which sourdough bread is made and would have to be carried through to totally eliminate gluten. A study confirmed that this resulted in bread that was not toxic to individuals with celiac disease (although the product resembled a biscuit more than a bread).

Bugs as Drugs—Hookworms

Our early contact with bacteria and toxins trains our immune systems. Based on the theory that as we have lost the chronic immune stimulation that came with all the infections mankind evolved with, parasites, including hookworms, are being ingested to stimulate the immune system in a protective way. This is a telling example of how much we need "bugs," and an exciting area of research. This approach has been used in Crohn's disease and asthma—using different kinds of parasites—and has been applied to celiac disease. The hookworms get in through the skin and travel to the intestinal tract via the bloodstream. They grow in the gut and exert an immune response.

One study showed no benefit, and another done recently did not reduce the severity of symptoms or prevent intestinal deterioration. But the parasitic infection did suppress some inflammatory responses, suggesting that further studies should be done.

Hookworms can cause anemia, and we do not recommend trying this approach at home—although they are often obtained unwittingly while on vacation in developing countries, where they are widespread.

Oral Passive Antibody Therapy

This approach has been considered for some time. The theory is that some animals can be immunized and produce antibodies to gluten. These antibodies can then be produced in sufficient quantities and administered to bind to gluten in the intestine. There are two proposed sources—one developed from the colostrum of cow's milk, and recently an antibody to gluten developed in hens' eggs. Individuals with an egg allergy could not take the latter product.

While the press releases of each new potential product attract much attention, there is a great deal of work to get a drug to market. It is an expensive and time-consuming project, and many products never make it to the shelf.

Probiotics

Probiotics are an exciting form of potential therapy. It is possible that they can be genetically enriched with drugs and then ingested into the small intestine, where they would release the potential drug at a needed site and act locally. However, much research needs to be done on this mode of therapy. Probiotics would have to move from the category of dietary supplement to that of a drug and thus undergo the rigorous safety and efficacy studies required for drugs to be sold in the U.S.

Over-the-Counter Drugs Currently Available

There are currently *no* products available over the counter that can fully degrade or digest gluten and block the effects it has on those with celiac disease, despite some manufacturers' claims to the contrary. Various OTC supplements are actively marketed in carefully worded advertisements that make claims about digesting gluten, healing the gut, and reducing inflammation. Manufacturers state in very fine print at the bottom of labels and websites that the supplements are not intended to cure or treat disease. And they advise people to take their products without the rigid testing for effectiveness and safety required by the FDA.

These products contain a variety of enzymes that can partially digest gluten in test tubes. However, studies by Dr. Frits Koning in the Netherlands have shown that they cannot digest gluten in the acidic environment of the stomach. In addition, they do not digest the toxic peptides that are resistant to the usual digestive enzymes. These different OTC supplements may also pose a health risk to anyone with undiagnosed celiac disease who believes they can "safely" eat gluten—all the while allowing it to silently inflame their intestines. We recommend that patients with celiac disease specifically avoid using these products as they could be harmful.

Most people with celiac disease and other GI disorders are careful about the foods they put in their mouth. They should be equally concerned—or even more careful—about OTC supplements they ingest.

FDA Approval

The development of therapies for celiac disease must follow a specific line negotiated by the drug companies with the FDA. Because celiac disease has specific tissue and biochemical abnormalities, it allows for the development of end points that must be satisfied prior to approval. These end points are agreed to prior to placebo-controlled studies. For celiac disease, therapies must prove to be effective in reducing inflammation and/or intestinal damage as well as symptoms. Most important, any drug must make people feel better. This needs to be determined in placebo-controlled randomized studies.

The FDA now also mandates that companies developing drugs develop a plan for studying the drug in children.

Once a drug is on the market, physicians can prescribe the medication for "off label" use to treat other conditions. It is anticipated that gluten-sensitive people may want these medications once they are available, especially if they are very sensitive to small amounts of gluten, as that is the target of the therapy. However, we hope to know more about gluten sensitivity and be able to target the cause—which may not be gluten, the gliadin fraction of wheat.

The Hazard of Taking a Pill

The widespread prescribing of statins (cholesterol-inhibiting drugs) has erroneously convinced some people that they can take a pill in the morning and then have a cheese omelet for lunch, "bread their butter," and then eat fried and creamed foods for dinner. They think, "The pill will take care of it." Statins can be "oversaturated" and essentially unable to take care of the cholesterol load ingested.

That is one of the real moral hazards of the new drugs being developed. Currently, they are not able to replace a gluten-free diet but do augment it and cover contamination or an occasional exposure. They are able to degrade small amounts of gluten, not a sandwich, pizza slices, or a piece of cake. People may take the medication and then feel it relieves them of the need to stay on a gluten-free diet. Or the medication may enable them to feel better when they eat out, all the while (unwittingly?) ingesting more gluten than the drug can handle. The patient then gets a low-grade chronic exposure to gluten for many years, feels good, does not get celiac-specific checkups, and develops a lymphoma in 10 years.

We will not find out how bad that may be for many people for decades, especially those who are asymptomatic—they can eat gluten and continue to have an immune inflammatory response and/or get the disease.

When choosing new treatment strategies, one must consider the possible risks versus benefits of the treatments against a gluten-free diet, which we know is safe, effectively eliminates the problem protein, and saves lives.

Questions Arise: Is the Drug Suitable for Me?

It is unclear if the drugs will work for everyone taking them. Some people might not respond and may not realize it. Other diseases or therapies could impact the delivery or efficacy of any of the potential therapies. For example, the enzymes that work in the stomach are dependent on an acidic environment—individuals cannot swallow acid blockers all the time and still have them work, and some people do not make acid at all (a condition known as hypochlorhydria).

Summary

There is a real need to continue to seek out and develop an alternative therapy to a gluten-free diet. Ideally, this will be a therapy that will not simply help with the diet by dealing with minor contamination, but that will allow people to eat a regular diet containing gluten.

Patients with celiac disease and most clinicians treating the patients will want to be convinced that any new drug for celiac disease is able to prevent the development of the gluten-induced damage to the lining of the small intestine, and ensure that patients live a long and symptom-free life.

The pipeline is built, but is not as yet pumping effective and safe treatments.

31

Eating Healthy

Don't eat anything your great-grandmother wouldn't recognize as food.
—MICHAEL POLLAN

*High-tech tomatoes. Mysterious milk. Supersquash. Are
we supposed to eat this stuff? Or is it going to eat us?*
—ANITA MANNING

Gluten is the most recent dietary sensation. But it is too often not a healthy one. Navigating your way to this particular table can be a dietary obstacle course.

The markets are filled with hidden gluten and, in gluten-free products, some ingredients that, for certain people, are possibly worse than gluten. There are also products and food manufacturing processes that may be contributing to the recent growth in celiac disease as well as other auto-immune conditions.

It is time to move the dialogue away from gluten alone and include everything else on your plate. We need to explore what is being done to gluten-free products to make them taste and look like the "real thing."

We may, in fact, be eating ourselves sick.

Emulsifiers, Binders, and Enhancers

In the Western world, most people who do not live on farms—growing and eating only what they produce—eat a diet of food that is processed to guard against spoilage, ensure longevity, and promote its taste and appeal. This includes everything from pasteurization (guarding against harmful bacteria) to supplementation with chemicals, vitamins, and minerals that put back what processing takes out—plus a list of sweeteners, salt, flavorings, and binders to make products more appealing to the perceived wants of the consumer.

Emulsifiers

They were like oil and water.
—PROVERBIAL PHRASE

Emulsifiers are a common additive used to stabilize food. For example, if you add oil to water and vigorously shake it, the oil will disperse throughout the water. Left to sit, the oil and water will separate. When you add an emulsifier, the oil stays dispersed and a stable emulsion is formed. Mustard will accomplish this for the oil and vinegar in a salad dressing; bile salts accomplish this in the intestine. They enable fats to be spread through the liquid contents of the intestine and be digested and absorbed into the body. Chemicals are used in food processing to hold products together.

Emulsions are found throughout the food industry. They are used in baking to form and maintain the volume and texture of biscuits and breads, and to improve the structure of crumbs in cakes. They are also in dairy products, confectionery items like chocolates and toffees, meats, margarine, and spreads (e.g., peanut butter).

A new study suggests that emulsifiers may be linked to metabolic syndrome and IBD. The study, reported in the academic journal *Nature*, showed that mice fed relatively low concentrations of two commonly used emulsifiers had low-grade inflammation and obesity/metabolic syndrome. The emulsifiers also promoted colitis in mice predisposed to this disorder. The researchers tested different species of bacteria in the mouse GI tract and hypothesized that a disruption of the microbiota encouraged the issues. While the scientists acknowledged that "excess caloric consumption was still a predominant factor driving the metabolic syndrome epidemic," the study pointed toward elements like emulsifiers in food as a potential promoter of low-grade intestinal inflammation.

If emulsifiers encourage inflammation in the gut, which in turn increases intestinal permeability ("leaky gut"), it would potentially enable food antigens and bacteria to move into the body from the intestinal tract, and might promote any number of allergies and conditions in predisposed people. More studies will need to be done to test this theory.

Food "Glue"

Another product used to enhance the texture and quality of food products is an enzyme called microbial transglutaminase (MTGase). It is a food "glue" that modifies proteins to improve the appearance, hardness, and shelf life of meat, the hardness of fish products, the quality and texture of milk and dairy products, the consistency and elasticity of candy, and the texture and volume of foods in commercially baked goods. If the label reads "added enzymes," those enzymes are more than likely MTGase.

Human tissue transglutaminase has long been recognized as the autoantigen of celiac disease—the enzyme that reacts with gliadin and sets off the reaction that triggers celiac disease. But transglutaminases are found throughout nature in mammal tissue, invertebrates, plants, and microbial cells. MTGase is the biological glue used in food products and some medicine. In fact, our diets may contain large amounts of MTGase, raising the question of its relation to the rise in incidences of celiac disease.

The key question is whether MTGase added to food increases the risk to those susceptible to celiac disease or nonceliac gluten sensitivity, or whether it can cause disease by itself in these individuals. While it is considered to be generally safe for the majority of people because it is approved as a natural product, several studies have led to the hypothesis that the industrial use of MTGase is a new environmental enhancer of celiac disease and may have negative effects on the gluten-sensitive population.

It does this in two ways. It may create toxic gluten peptides capable of producing an immune response prior to ingestion; and/or once eaten, these peptides may increase toxicity in the intestine and initiate celiac disease in susceptible individuals.

MTGase is also used on gluten-free ingredients (e.g., soy) in gluten-free products. Thus a product labeled "gluten-free" but containing soy that has been cross-linked using MTGase creates an additional layer of confusion. Gluten-free foods frequently and inevitably contain small amounts of gluten, and these small amounts of contaminants would become more toxic to people with celiac disease due to MTGase action.

The scientists studying MTGase concluded that "If future research substantiates this hypothesis, the findings will affect food product labeling, food additive policies of the food industry, and consumer health education."

It is something to think about when you reach for processed products in the market. Because MTGase is not a food, it is not required to be listed on food labels.

Vital Gluten

For those who are focused solely on the gluten in their food, it is available in industrial-strength form.

Vital gluten is a powdered form of the protein portion of wheat with the starch washed out. It is sold alongside many flours and advertised as a "natural," "high-protein" baking product that improves the texture and elasticity of dough. One manufacturer advertises it as something that "can easily put the home bread baker on a par with the professionals." It is not a flour but powdered gluten.

Vital wheat gluten is the main ingredient in seitan, a food product used in vegetarian cooking and often referred to as "wheat meat." Wheat gluten is also used as a source of protein and in pet foods as a binder. Wheat gluten from China, adulterated by melamine, was blamed as the cause of pet food recalls in 2007. It also can hold other food products together, e.g., mushroom or vegetarian burgers.

It is unclear what effect a vegetarian or vegan diet high in vital wheat gluten might have on someone with a genetic susceptibility to celiac disease. Researchers are examining this issue.

Are You Eating Products or Food?

While nondairy milk may be of value for individuals who are lactose intolerant or dedicated to a vegan diet, it is not a food. Milk is a natural product of lactation, not of an electric blender or manufacturing plant. Juices that claim to have "fresh from the orange" taste often do not have fresh-from-the-orange ingredients.

Labels are required to list all ingredients in descending order by amount. If the first ingredient is water, then there is more water in the product than anything else. If we break down the label on soy or almond milk, both consist mainly of water that is sweetened and supplemented with calcium, vitamins, and thickening agents.

Both soy and almond milk usually contain carrageenan (highly processed seaweed), added to create a creamy texture—and implicated in inflammation and GI problems.

All these labels boast "natural" vitamins. Vitamins are found in all of the foods we eat—that is the natural form. Added vitamins are manufactured (calcium carbonate, D2, vitamin-synthetic vitamin A) and often lack the cofactors (the other food and/or vitamins) necessary for them to be properly absorbed by the body.

Adding back vitamins after the fact ignores the issue of synergy: how nutrients work naturally as opposed to when they are isolated. A 2011 study on broccoli at the Linus Pauling Institute illustrates this point. The researchers found that giving subjects fresh broccoli florets led them to absorb and metabolize seven times more of the anticancer compounds known as glucosinolates, present in broccoli and other cruciferous vegetables (Brussels sprouts, collard greens, kale) than when glucosinolates were given in straight capsule form. The researchers hypothesized that this might be because the fresh broccoli contained other compounds that helped people's bodies put the broccoli's anticancer chemicals to use.

There is a certain amount of irony in the instructions to take vitamins and certain minerals (i.e., calcium) with food for proper digestion and bodily effectiveness. Supplementation is also ironically praiseworthy as it returns to the food supply all the natural vitamins and minerals food processing and our diets have taken out.

Everyone on a gluten-free diet should try to eat and drink less processed food. Your symptoms may be coming from ingredients that sound natural but are actually intestinal irritants.

Where Is Gluten Hiding?

Gluten is found not only in products made with wheat, rye, and barley, but as an ingredient to modify texture, facilitate water or fat retention, and help bind products, from soups and meats to ready-to-eat meals, etc. It is also used as a filler in drug and supplement capsules.

In accordance with the FDA labeling law passed in 2013, any food labeled gluten-free must contain "less than 20mg/kg gluten" (less than 20 parts per million). The ruling further specifies that any "foods specially processed to reduce gluten content" or "very low gluten" must comply with levels between 20 and 100 mg/kg.

This is a controversial area, as there are different tests used by manufacturers to determine gluten content, and testing batches in food products varies. Since the labeling process is voluntary, there is no government-regulated testing to confirm labeling in the U.S. as there is in Canada. A few studies have shown contamination of gluten-free foods and medications/supplements, even in those made of inherently gluten-free grains.

Cross-Contamination

Cross-contamination can occur at any level of food production. While this problem is mainly directed to people with celiac disease who require a truly gluten-free product to maintain their health, there are few guarantees in place.

A number of so-called gluten-free flours and grains actually have tested for unsafe levels of contamination. Many home cooks can find the source of digestive problems related to gluten within their stock of gluten-free ingredients. Manufacturers may also receive batches of contaminated grains while making products in a dedicated facility. Unless they do regular on-site testing using validated assays, this can be an issue.

While various experts have studied the contamination of oats with wheat and barley, it is not the only grain that can be contaminated. Other grains that are naturally gluten-free, like millet, have been shown to be frequently contaminated by wheat.

To guarantee that a grain is gluten-free, it needs to be either grown and processed in dedicated fields and facilities, or, alternatively, tested to be free of gluten. All grains except for rice also have to be labeled "gluten-free" because of contamination studies.

Bulk Bins

Contamination can occur when food is displayed in open bins in the market. Suzanne Simpson, R.D., warns patients not to buy from bulk bins with a scoop. Scoops "travel" and can find themselves in the raisin bin having started the morning in another nearby bin containing a product with gluten. She also warns patients to beware of websites selling nuts, flours, and mixes that must be carefully monitored to be safe.

Reading Labels

You can fool all the people some of the time, and some of the people all the time, but you cannot fool all the people all the time.
—ABRAHAM LINCOLN

We came up with a system. If the label has more than three different things that you cannot pronounce, then it's not really good for you.

(OWEN, 12)

If you are trying to be gluten-free, you need to read labels to avoid gluten. But many foods require no stamp of approval, as they are naturally gluten-free. Water is at the top of the list, yet there are actually water bottles labeled "gluten-free" and selling at a premium—"because you can never be too sure." Labeling rules now allow water as well as other products to be labeled gluten-free even though they may be just that by nature. The only thing that this label likely ensures is that you are paying more money unnecessarily.

The foods that require a gluten-free label are anything made from or with flours: cereals, pastas, breads, cookies, cakes, pretzels, rice cakes, crackers, pizza, breaded and frozen items, etc. Soups, mixes, and all-in-one products with packets of flavorings (e.g., rice pilaf mixes) should also be scrutinized carefully.

While there are many forms of hidden gluten, if a product contains wheat in any of its forms, it must be listed on the label. Barley is not part of the labeling law and must be identified in its various forms (malt) and uses (beer).

Reading labels is important and not difficult once certain words are ruled out. For example, malt is made from barley, but when it is the first four letters in a long word such as *maltodextrin* or *maltitol* it is safe. Yeast as an ingredient is fine, but brewer's yeast is not.

If a product is made in a facility that processes other products with wheat—and is not labeled gluten-free—it may be contaminated. If it is labeled gluten-free, it is most likely safe.

Eating Healthy

Despite the many roadblocks, the road to a healthy gluten-free diet can be found by focusing on minimally processed foods that are naturally nutrient rich.

If you decide to go on a gluten-free diet—or are already following one—there are some basic principles to follow.

- Eat a *balanced* and *varied* diet that is high in whole foods and low in manufactured food products.
- Eat plenty of fresh fruits and vegetables.
- Add more whole grains that are gluten-free and high in fiber (quinoa, amaranth, corn, buckwheat, millet).
- Eat raw and "crunchy" cooked vegetables as well as beans and foods with skin to get as much soluble fiber as possible.
- Eat plenty of protein from various sources (fish, lean meat and poultry, beans, seeds, and nuts).

- Eat gluten-free products that are high in sugar and fat sparingly.
- Avoid processed products with long ingredient lists (they usually contain excessive chemical additives).

A healthy diet is not accomplished on a 7- or 14-day plan. It is a long-term commitment to changing bad habits and eating differently.

A Note on Adding Fiber

A gluten-free diet doesn't mean living on rice, corn, and potatoes. I use as little of those ingredients as possible in my baking and daily diet. Instead, I rely on my good friends, the great gluten-free whole grains and flours like buckwheat, quinoa, oats, amaranth, sorghum, chickpea, and teff. You only have to look at their nutritional profiles to see that each one is a powerhouse of nutrients, fiber, and protein. I rely on these to add back some protein and elasticity to my baking, thus improving texture and structure. For best results in baking, add 25 to 30 percent to a flour blend. These flours are more finely ground and do not impart the unpleasant grittiness that often accompanies rice flour. No wonder I call them my best friends!

—BETH HILLSON, FOOD EDITOR, *GLUTEN FREE & MORE*, AUTHOR OF *GLUTEN-FREE MAKEOVERS*

All grains, whether gluten-free or not, contain fiber. Quinoa, oats, and lentils are especially high in fiber, and unless you're accustomed to a high-fiber diet, the fiber by itself can cause symptoms. Whenever a patient with IBS symptoms or celiac disease has a flare of symptoms and says that they are "trying to eat really healthy," it often means they have increased their fiber and have not tolerated the rapid increase. Their problem may also be an intolerance to fructose or other FODMAPs.

If you are trying to eat healthier and add grains, fresh fruit, and vegetables rapidly, be careful not to confuse the possible ensuing bloating with a return of symptoms.

Summary

- A healthy gluten-free diet is one of variety and filled with "food" rather than "products" made from ingredients grown in a lab and compiled in a manufacturing plant.
- Substitute wisely—adding too many sugar- and fat-filled gluten-free cakes, cookies, and snacks will add pleasure, but also pounds.
- Be smart when reading labels. "Natural" does not mean healthy.
- Diversify your diet—try new grains, vegetables, and fruits.
- Removing gluten from your diet may be a lifesaver, a symptom reliever, or a road to continuing medical issues. Eating gluten-free and eating healthy are not synonymous.

32

Myths and Misconceptions

Fables should be taught as fables, myths as myths, and miracles as poetic fantasies. To teach superstitions as truths is a most terrible thing.
—HYPATIA

Myths are widely held ideas that are false. But studies show that the more you tell people they are wrong, the more they believe their deeply held ideas. The following myths are a combination of "the usual suspects"—myths about gluten that absolutely refuse to die—and some interesting new misconceptions and questions that surround gluten.

Gluten causes dementia and Alzheimer's.

No, it does not. These two conditions are not related to gluten. Some of the symptoms of the "brain fog" that many patients describe can be confused for the early stages of these conditions, but brain fog is a discrete entity.

Gluten causes "brain fog," and a gluten-free diet can boost brainpower and improve mental focus.

Although brain fog is a poorly defined medical condition, it is frequently reported by patients. A medical term that encompasses this may well be "mild cognitive impairment." In recently diagnosed patients with celiac disease, studies show brain fog is common, but it improves with a gluten-free diet (and with the healing of the small intestine). There are no studies involving people with gluten sensitivity, nor is there any concrete science that indicates gluten causes brain fog in the general population.

There have also been no scientific studies that have shown that eliminating gluten from your diet (again, in the general population—and not those with celiac disease or a gluten-related issue) can boost your brainpower, improve mental focus, or prevent a decline in memory. (See chapter 28 for a more detailed discussion.)

Also, one could make an argument that thinking your focus is better makes it so—part of the placebo effect. And stomach issues in general, such as gas, bloating, and pain can decrease one's ability to concentrate. A feeling of fatigue or sleepiness after a meal may well be normal and related to hormones produced in the intestine. There are many studies that are exploring a brain-gut interaction but there is much that is unknown and several hypotheses that need to be explored before these claims can be substantiated.

Eating gluten makes you fat.

Eating more calories than you can burn off during your daily activities will add pounds to your body. A diet that contains grains will not, in itself, make you fat. The amount you eat will determine your weight.

Gluten-free baked goods and snacks contain high amounts of sugar and fat to enhance their taste and hold them together. On a gluten-free diet, patients often gain weight when they substitute these gluten-free foods for their wheat-based counterparts.

A gluten-free diet is healthier.

Unless you have a specific food allergy or intolerance, or a disease requiring food restrictions, a diverse diet—one that includes meat-based foods, dairy, fats, fresh fruits, vegetables, and whole grains that are high in fiber—is the healthiest. (See chapter 31, "Eating Healthy.")

Everyone should try eating gluten-free for a week.

While a week of gluten-free eating is generally harmless, the majority of people have nothing to gain. You are also removing a great deal of fiber, vitamins, and minerals from your diet and need to replace them with plenty of fruits, vegetables, and other grains. Studies have also confirmed that a trial gluten-free diet is not a test for celiac disease.

The fact that something is harmless does not mean it is good for you. This is an adjunct to the concept that something labeled "natural" is therefore harmless. All plants are natural, but many are highly toxic.

Is gluten sensitivity common?

Since medical science does not know how to define or test for gluten sensitivity, it is unclear how prevalent it may be. A recent double-blind study showed that only about 30 percent of people who believed they were "gluten sensitive" actually had adverse reactions when fed gluten. The condition is real, but it is not believed to be as widespread as some experts report. There are many other causes of GI symptoms that people blame on gluten alone.

Is there a gene test for gluten sensitivity?

There is no genetic link to nonceliac gluten sensitivity and therefore no gene test that is meaningful.

Can you diagnose celiac disease with just a blood test?

Blood tests are the first step used to determine if someone has celiac disease. If they are positive, the next steps are an endoscopy and biopsy. The results of a biopsy are still the gold standard for diagnosis.

There are strict guidelines followed by some physicians in Europe that use only blood tests to diagnosis children, but this standard has not been accepted in the U.S.

A complete listing of tests for celiac disease, as well as a fuller discussion of this issue, can be found in chapters 6 and 17.

Does corn raise celiac antibody levels?

Corn is not harmful for the majority of people with celiac disease. But some individuals have corn allergies or sensitivities as a separate issue. So you can have celiac disease *and* IgE antibodies (allergy based) to corn. Eating corn will not increase your antibodies to gluten.

Can gluten pass through the skin?

Gliadin is not absorbed through the skin, but it can enter the GI tract through the more porous mucous membranes of the nose and mouth. Therefore, lipstick can be a source of gluten. You can also breathe it in.

The skin barrier is designed to keep the outside world out—but if your skin is broken or damaged, gluten can get through. But it will not cause dermatitis herpetiformis (the skin manifestation of celiac disease).

Gluten can worsen hives, canker sores, psoriasis, and eczema in some people. There are also numerous ingredients in lotions and shampoos that can cause skin irritation and inflammation, which may then be blamed on gluten in the product.

What does it mean when antibodies to different foods are found in the stool?

Very little. We do not know how commonly antibodies to foods occur in those with no symptoms. Stool tests are not a reliable test for allergies or celiac disease.

Does having celiac disease mean that my immune system is depressed or suppressed?

No, it is just the opposite—it is more active. The gluten-free diet removes the trigger activating the immune system and causing the inflammation.

This is one reason that people with undiagnosed but active celiac disease are more likely to develop a second autoimmune condition: their immune systems are overactive, and can turn against the body.

There are, however, specific instances in which the immune system can be compromised—people with active celiac disease have impaired spleen function. The mechanism of this is not clear. Since pneumococcal and meningococcal bacteria require normal spleen function to be cleared by humans, it is recommended that individuals with celiac disease receive a pneumococcal vaccination.

There is evidence that those with celiac disease who fail to follow a gluten-free diet are at greater risk of developing more autoimmune diseases than those who do adhere to it. It is another reason that people with celiac disease are well advised to follow a strict gluten-free diet.

Over-the-counter (OTC) enzymes containing DPP4 "digest" gluten.

There are currently *no* OTC products that are able to digest the toxic fractions of gluten. Most of the "enzymes" found in these products (DPP4, amylase) are already found in the intestinal tract, where they are not able to break down the complex gliadin protein. Many people do not realize that they are paying money for OTC products containing ingredients claiming to digest gluten that are already present in the body and unable to do the job.

You can outgrow celiac disease.

Celiac disease is an autoimmune condition that cannot be outgrown. Some people do not have overt symptoms after eating gluten and may think this means they have outgrown it. But even without symptoms, the grain may be silently inflaming their intestines and causing an autoimmune reaction throughout the body that will manifest in more serious disease years later. (This topic is discussed in more detail in chapter 17.)

Genetically modified wheat is causing the rise in celiac disease and gluten-related disorders today.

Wheat today has been genetically modified by regular cultivation practices of crossbreeding to produce species with a higher yield that contain more protein and carbohydrates than the strains of wild grains found 10,000 years ago. The various species of wheat available today each contain different flavors, qualities, and uses (bread, pasta, cakes, etc.). In addition, some flours are fortified with "vital wheat gluten" to enhance their baking properties. This may contribute to increasing the gluten content of wheat products and the development of celiac disease. (See chapter 17, "Celiac Disease.")

Nevertheless, the modification of wheat cannot explain the rise in gluten-related disorders and celiac disease. In fact, it has been scientifically linked to many more environmental factors beyond wheat itself. These include the rise in antibiotic and other drug use—both OTC and prescription—that may alter the intestinal balance of microbiota living there, the hygiene hypothesis (see chapter 3, "Picky Eaters"), and possibly the change in diet to more processed food that is chemically enriched, preserved and pasteurized (see chapter 4, "Pitfalls and Perils of a Gluten-Free Diet") and other individual genetic, age, health, and lifestyle factors.

Researchers have been examining wheat species for the past two decades to try to isolate cultivars (specifically bred strains) of wheat that may be less and/or nontoxic to people with celiac disease and gluten sensitivity. In addition, there are attempts to genetically modify wheat in the laboratory (GMO wheat). At this point in time, it is unclear if any of these genetically modified wheat species that lack the toxic aspects of gluten can compete with regular wheat in terms of taste, baking and cooking qualities, and yield. But stay tuned.

Thus, wheat modification is neither cause nor *currently* a cure for gluten-related disorders.

Glyphosates are contributing to the dramatic increase in celiac disease.

Glyphosate is the active ingredient in the herbicide Roundup. It is an herbicide whose extensive use has led to an increase in weeds resistant to the product. This has become a serious problem for farmers, and therefore other products were developed to handle these weeds, leading the EPA to place restrictions on the levels of these herbicides allowable in water.

One paper became the banner for the antiglyphosate movement when it stated that glyphosate was a key contributor to the obesity and autism epidemics in the U.S., as well as to Alzheimer's disease, Parkinson's disease, infertility, depression, cancer, and celiac disease.

A number of scientists at Monsanto, the maker of Roundup, found the paper to be "a collection of unrelated data points that drew conclusion from observations that were incorrect or poorly established." In fact, the study was a collection of assertions that were not backed up by the observations cited. But the disapproval then went well beyond the Monsanto review of the paper when numerous other scientists and science writers joined the debate.

They saw "bad science becoming truth online" and posted an article "When Media Uncritically Cover Pseudoscience." One writer called "this kind of alarmism unethical and irresponsible."

While it is becoming increasingly apparent that the many chemicals we put in our food—to grow, enlarge, and/or bind it, in addition to those to make it taste better (especially the "low-fat" varieties)—may be harming us in unknown ways, association is not cause. Whether glyphosate is toxic to more than weeds is scientifically questionable. And whether it somehow epigenetically affects the genome is intriguing, but also unproven.

Can you drink coffee if you have celiac disease?

Regular and decaffeinated coffee are gluten-free. Flavored coffees and coffee drinks may contain gluten—check the label, especially for sweeteners with malt. Instant, ground, or whole-bean coffee should be gluten-free, but again, check the label. Flavoring can add ingredients that are not gluten-free.

The only vodka that is safe to drink, i.e., gluten-free, is made from potatoes.

All distilled spirits are safe for people with celiac disease to drink. The gliadin molecule is removed during distillation. If "distillate" is added back or flavorings are added that are not distilled and contain gluten, these vodkas would not be safe to drink.

Fermented alcohols made of grain, such as beer, are not gluten-free, as the fermentation process does not remove the gluten.

And saving the best for last:

I read it on the Internet (so it must be true).

Medical misinformation is widely available on the Internet and in the popular press. If you search hard enough, you will eventually find a "doctor" or post to tell you what you want to hear.

If you are searching the web, make sure you look into the background of the person writing the piece. This holds true for any book or article you read. The ability to use buzzwords and medical terms does not mean someone is an expert on the subject or capable of giving you good advice. Many articles and so-called "medical" sites that are not affiliated with major medical centers are way ahead of the science and often misleading. If someone claims to be an expert, check them out on PubMed. This is where scientific articles and true expertise reside.

If you are looking for answers to your symptoms, you should make an appointment with a medical doctor.

33

Food for Thought

Stories Matter: Different Roads to a Healthy Life

I had horrible stomach problems my entire life and no one could tell me what was wrong. I had horrible diarrhea and a lot of vomiting, and no one knew what that was from. People gave me various diagnoses, from milk allergies to "neurotic and stressed out," that kind of stuff. No one ever could say what was wrong.

I was at my OB-GYN and she said, "You're really deficient in iron and a lot of other things—you should go to a gastroenterologist and be tested for celiac disease." So I did and he said, "It's very unlikely: you don't look like someone who would have celiac disease." So I went to another doctor who did a blood test and found [high] antibodies, then did an endoscopy and found pretty severe damage. I was diagnosed with celiac disease almost 10 years ago.

In the beginning I was a lot more paranoid and nervous about it—I didn't want to go to restaurants at all and made everything for myself. I would scrutinize labels and was incredibly restrictive. And there was also so much less out there.

Now I feel more comfortable. Restaurants are more educated about it. But if I am exposed to anything with gluten, my reaction is much, much worse. I have horrible, unbearable headaches for days that nothing can help.

The only time it's stressful is when I'm going to a business lunch or something honoring someone and there are 500 people. I'm never sure if I'll show up at a large function and there'll be nothing to eat. Sometimes I would eat before and not say anything.

I think now people don't take it as seriously as before because of all the new fads with dieting. Now when I say to people, "I can't eat gluten," there's some eye-rolling—like, "Oh, she's one of those women who has weird food fixations." Which is kind of annoying because it trivializes the disease and how serious it is.

The hardest part is having a child who doesn't have celiac disease. He spreads crumbs with gluten everywhere, puts his hand in my mouth. That has been a challenge and has made me sick a few times.

In the great scheme of things, it's not that bad. I'd only advise people to be very careful about the diet. I would tell them how much better I felt once I was diagnosed.

(ANNABELLE, 33)

I went on a gluten-free diet at the suggestion of my gastroenterologist. I have what they call idiopathic irritable bowel syndrome—which means they can't figure out what's causing my symptoms, but I've got a litany of them. My mom also had a terrible digestive system; she always had indigestion.

I get constipated for two to three days, and my colon fills and presses on my bladder. So I have to urinate frequently. When you have to hold that much fecal matter, your back hurts. I couldn't get comfortable until I had a bowel movement. But I was constipated and couldn't go. So I took medicine to poop and got diarrhea and took medicine to stop. The doctor said, "You've got to stop taking all these drugs to go and stop." And when it finally moves through the last part there is *major* discomfort getting it out.

And the gas—I can literally see my belly blow up. I get bloated for two to three days and look like I'm four months pregnant. It's not gas that I can eliminate—it just sits there; it's this grumble. I also have something where the vaginal wall is falling—I think it's called pelvic floor dysfunction—which adds to these symptoms. My gynecologist suggested that I eat more fiber and change my diet.

My internist knew all the issues and suggested I change my diet by cutting back on carbs. I finally went on a gluten-free diet when my gastroenterologist said that gluten or something might be causing an issue in my digestion system and I should try the gluten-free diet and see if that helped. He tested me for celiac disease, and that was negative. He also put me on Linzess to loosen the fecal matter—after I had tried every other pill on the market so the insurance company would allow it.

I don't go crazy about the diet—I do not have to worry if I've had something with gluten so some may be in my diet. I read labels and understand hidden gluten. I don't eat packaged things and have never been a big bread eater anyway. I'm always happy with potatoes; I've never met one I didn't like.

This combination of things has made a difference. I don't have terrible gas pains and bloating and the difficulty of having fecal matter move through my body. There's no weight loss, none of that. I cook and I bake. What I've learned in my 53 years—everything in moderation.

I think it has made a big difference. Everyone comes to it from a different perspective. And this works for me.

(CASSIE, 53)

The reason I went on a gluten-free diet? I have Graves' disease [hyperthyroidism]. I had a terribly bad reaction—pounding heart, my hair fell out. I've been on and off different levels of methimazole [to control symptoms], but you can't take that forever. The flares, which were quite severe, responded to the drug the first two times. The third flare was mild, but I still needed medicine. After that episode, I asked my doctor: "Could diet play a part in this?" She said no.

But I believe, I really do believe, that being on a gluten-free diet helps to control these symptoms—these racing thyroid levels. Looking back, I do associate eating barley and pizza with an awful lot of bloating. I have not been able to digest barley for years. I get quite a sore belly. But I've never been tested for celiac disease. After the third episode I went gluten-free, and I've been symptom free for the past two to three years. And just in general I think I feel better.

(MAURI, 62)

For everyone calling me anorexic—I have a gluten and lactose allergy. It's not about weight; it's about health. Gluten is crapppp anyway!

—MILEY CYRUS, ON TWITTER

Everyone comes to a gluten-free diet with his or her own story—celiac disease, gastrointestinal and/or neurological symptoms, psychiatric conditions, or simply interest in the latest dietary "cure." People who avoid wheat and gluten are often seen as an aggregate, but they are in fact a diverse group of individuals who must find different roads to a healthy life.

There is rarely one simple solution—such as eliminating grains or gluten—no matter how appealing that may be, and not every symptom can be readily resolved. It is possible that some of the answers may lie at the very core of our individuality—in our genes and the ecosystem of microbiota living in our guts, or how each of our brains perceive and react to illness.

What Is Making Us Sick—Gluten or Genetics Gone Awry?

Our individuality begins with our genome and, also important, how each of us reacts to our environments. There is a great deal of variety between the responses of people to the same environmental risk, which implies that genetic susceptibility may play a big role in certain diseases. Celiac disease requires specific genes, as do autoimmune conditions such as type 1 diabetes, other common diseases such as hypertension, or congenital conditions such as cleft palate.

Our genes/DNA are an instruction manual for every cell in the body—they send directions for cells to be skin or bone, hair to be red or black or brown, the cholesterol produced in your liver to be high or low. They are the underlying source code for body function—and perhaps its disrepair.

A key question is whether certain genes that originally evolved as a protective measure to fight infections, i.e., involved in survival, are now putting people at risk for other conditions. While the original function has become obsolete, the gene remains and is now reacting to the current environment. New genetic research is expanding our knowledge of why so many more people have celiac disease and a host of related autoimmune disorders. And the environment may also be rewriting the DNA instruction manual.

Epigenetics

Epigenetics is a term coined in 1942 to describe alterations in the expression or behavior of a gene caused by environmental factors. These changes do not affect the underlying DNA, but exist "on top of" (*epi*, Greek) the genetic inheritance.

If the DNA instruction manual arrives at the cell with directions in Chinese, and the cell can only read English, the gene would be silenced, unable to read the instructions. And if the manual contained faulty instructions, the cell's behavior would be altered accordingly.

In this way the epigenetic environmental changes do not affect the DNA of the gene but only how it behaves and may be altering how the body responds. If the environment can modify gene expression through epigenetic mechanisms, it may contribute to autoimmune disease in a genetically predisposed person. It has been proven that epigenetic dysregulation plays a role in cancer, and researchers are exploring the effect it may have on diet-related chronic diseases such as type 2 diabetes, obesity, cardiovascular disease, and perhaps celiac disease.

The influence of environment is particularly important during our development and may induce permanent changes in bodily structure, gene expression, and disease risk. If someone becomes sensitized to foods during early development, the effect may last into adulthood.

Or Is It Genes and Germs?

If humans are a composite of microbial and human cells, the human genetic landscape becomes an aggregate of the genes in the human genome and the microbiome—a blend of human and microbial traits. Understanding this immense diversity and the factors affecting it is one of the main goals of a new initiative—the Human Microbiome Project (HMP). The HMP is looking to identify and characterize the microorganisms found in both healthy and diseased humans.

Because the microbiome is populated vertically (genetically) as well as horizontally (by the environment) it may be that our genes determine the composition of our microbiome, thereby predisposing it to disease susceptibility.

Many studies are now showing that changes in the composition of our microbiome correlate with various disease states, raising the possibility that manipulating our bacterial friends and foes may be a way to treat disease.

It may be possible that the newest keys to health will not be an alteration in our diets, but in the bacteria that feeds on it.

How Great Is the Placebo Effect?

Responding to a gluten-free diet does not indicate gluten sensitivity. The response could be a placebo or nocebo effect.

The placebo effect (*placebo* is Latin for "I shall please") is a well-studied and well-known phenomenon in which a dummy treatment or therapy creates a beneficial response simply because the person taking it feels that it will help. In various studies, sugar pills often produce the same result as actual drugs.

While the exact psychological and neurological explanation of why inactive placebos work as well as the active drug in different trials is still unclear, various hypotheses (pills reduce anxiety, modulate expectations, raise self-awareness and attention) have been suggested. This has also been studied in alternative medicine, where rituals may act as a placebo.

Nocebo (Latin for "I shall harm") is a substance or therapy that creates a harmful effect. The responses are a result of the patient's perception of how the substance will affect him or her. A nocebo creates the perception that a substance will be harmful, and these negative expectations can create an actual symptom. In one study of lactose intolerance, people were told they were receiving lactose but were in fact receiving a glucose pill. A large percentage of people with lactose intolerance (44 percent) and without (26 percent) complained of GI symptoms. Often, when doctors tell patients of the side effects of a drug or therapy—which they are ethically required to do—there is an increased likelihood that the patient will experience the side effect. People anticipating the negative effects of gluten can actually feel symptoms. The placebo and nocebo responses are another reason the FDA requires double-blind studies in which both the patient and the researcher are not aware of who is getting the active drug.

The mind is a powerful tool. Believing something is bad or good for you can make it so. Studies on the actual versus believed effects of gluten on various groups show this to be the case, perhaps contributing to the "glutenitis" surge reported in the media.

Gluten Realities

We have stopped natural selection from purifying
the species because deep in our heart of hearts, we
are all terrified that we won't make the cut.
—MOXIE MEZCAL, WRITER

A gluten-free diet is many things.

It is a miracle treatment if you have celiac disease.

It is a myth if you think that eliminating gluten it is a healthy or effective weight-loss diet, or that it causes every brain or gut condition in the medical textbooks.

It is a menace if you eat the many gluten-free foods and supplements that contain heavy metals and potentially dangerous binders and emulsions.

Natural selection has given way to antibiotics, stents, and statins, and a focus on pills and potions that supposedly give us a biological advantage. We all want answers and our "connected world" promises that they are all readily available, but many of the substances we ingest to outwit Mother Nature may not be the clever strategies we think them to be.

With any new therapy there is often a great wave of enthusiasm that settles down to an appropriate level. To be of proven value any medical treatment needs time. The FODMAP diet is a good example of this. Irritable bowel syndrome is so difficult to manage in many patients that the early reports of great success with this diet caused a lot of enthusiastic support. Current studies showing a much lower rate of resolved symptoms are dampening that enthusiasm. But as with any therapy, the FODMAP diet will find its place as placebo-controlled studies on it are done.

The results of another large study on the effect of breast-feeding and the early introduction of gluten as a means of controlling celiac disease has recently been shown to be incorrect. This changes a decade of advice to patients. Again, it required a placebo-controlled study!

Isolate, Test First, Treat Right

There is a great deal of talk about "personalized medicine." This has various meanings that include matching treatment/drugs to a patient's genes (or those of a tumor or cell) as well as their characteristics, needs, and preferences. We look at personalized medicine as the basis of good doctoring—helping each patient navigate his or her own road to health. Gluten has a place in medical treatment—but it must be part of an individual story. Gluten is simply not causing the many conditions it is blamed for—nor can it treat and cure them. Test first—before going on a gluten-free diet.

As scientists uncover the mysteries of our brains, guts, and microbiota, new treatments and solutions will be found, and some old remedies will undoubtedly regain importance or fall by the wayside. Gluten will eventually find its scientific place.

You cannot put the same shoe on every foot.
—PUBLILIUS SYRUS

Diets Through the Ages

Diets have been practiced since the beginning of time—not always by choice.

Approximately 150,000 BC—The Neanderthal (aka Paleo) Diet

Lacking an abundance of food, Neanderthals ate whatever they could hunt or forage. Luck meant a mammoth or small deer, but their protein was limited and they had periods of near starvation. Despite the "paleofantasy" of the raw food diet, Neanderthals ate both cooked and raw meats as well as foraged tubers, plants, wild grains, and fruits.

Approximately 10,000 BC—Agriculture Arrives

Cultivated grains were added to the diet during the agricultural revolution, but wild grains were part of the early human diet before that.

Ancient Greeks and Romans—The Original Mediterranean Diet

Mens sana in corpore sana—a healthy mind in a healthy body.

The Ancient Greeks and Romans left records of weight loss diets. Prescriptions for weight loss included vomiting, purgation (enema or laxative), worry, hard beds, heat, vigorous exercise, and eating sour and harsh things. Sour foods were often tainted or bad, which circled back to vomiting . . .

Pliny the Elder based his dietary advice on wine. To gain weight, drink wine with meals; to lose it, avoid wine with meals.

Middle Ages—Anti-Sin Diets

Some of the first diets came from the religious crusades against sin. Gluttony was one of the seven deadly sins, and hermits and monks seeking to cleanse mind and body ate a normal diet for five days and fasted for two.

Saint Catherine of Siena denied herself food as part of the spiritual denial of self.

People in the Middle Ages were also known to binge and purge in order to eat more at a meal. Now this is called bulimia.

Circa 1829—Vegetarian Diet

Sylvester Graham, an ordained preacher and dietary reformer, created the first vegetarian diet. Consisting mainly of fruits, vegetables, whole wheat, and high-fiber foods, limited amounts of milk products and eggs, and no meat or spices, the diet was believed to prevent "impure thought and in turn . . . stop masturbation," which Graham believed to cause blindness and early death. Graham is known more for the cracker named after him, a staple of the diet.

Circa 1850s—The First Low-Carb Diet

William Harvey treated English undertaker William Banting for obesity. Based on a diabetes management regime he had learned about in Paris, Harvey advised Banting to cut down on sugars and starches. This appears to be the first low-carb diet.

Circa Late 1800s—The Chew and/or Spit Diet

William Gladstone, Britain's prime minister, advised that food must be chewed 32 times before swallowed. The theory was based on the principle that the chewing could lessen one's appetite, which would lead to weight loss. By the turn of the 20th century, Horace Fletcher advocated the "chew and spit" diet, which recommended chewing food until all the "goodness" was extracted and then spitting the rest out. Now this is called an eating disorder.

Early 1900s—The Tapeworm Diet

Although later credited to opera singer Maria Callas, the tapeworm diet involves swallowing a parasite-packed pill (or live parasites). Side effects include weight gain (those worms are hungry), pain, nausea, malnutrition, vitamin deficiencies, diarrhea, and weakness. Tapeworms can grow up to 30 feet.

1918—The Calorie Goes Mainstream

Wilbur Atwater, an American chemist, discovered the energy provided by food and its caloric value in the late 1880s. It was not until 1918 that the concept went mainstream, when Dr. Lulu Hunt Peters wrote a best-seller that outlined the first methods of counting calories as a method to lose weight. Dr. Peters outlined 100-calorie portions of different foods and espoused counting calories to regulate weight.

1925—The Cigarette Diet

Lucky Strike cigarettes introduce the "Reach for a Lucky instead of a sweet" campaign, which promoted nicotine's ability to suppress appetite.

1930s—The Grapefruit Diet

This diet required eating grapefruit with every meal. It claimed that grapefruit had fat-burning enzymes or properties. It was normally consumed with high-fat foods. It was not until many decades later that the harmful effect of grapefruit interacting with numerous drugs came to light.

1950s—The Cabbage Soup Diet

This quick weight loss diet was based on consuming as much cabbage soup as you want every day with a limited amount of other foods. Most of the weight lost on this radical short-term diet is water. It created a great deal of interest and flatulence.

Circa 1960—Macrobiotic Arrives

The Zen or macrobiotic diet is a grain-heavy approach credited to Christoph Wilhelm Hufeland, a German doctor, and Sagen Ishizuka, a Japanese military doctor. The Japanese-style diet varies from the Western one, but both rely on whole grains, especially rice, vegetables, beans, legumes, and naturally processed foods. Fish and seafood, seeds and nuts, and fruits and beverages are allowed several times a week. Highly processed and refined foods are avoided, as are most animal products.

1963—Weight Watchers

Weight Watchers, founded by Jean Nidetch, is based on restricting consumption to approximately 1,000 calories per day until an optimal weight is achieved, but all foods are allowed. The group offers meetings, support material, and tracking tools to allow "members" to track their personal calorie deficits and stay on course. Dieters are given social support as well as dietary advice.

1970s and 1980s—Drugs and Appetite Suppressants

The appetite suppressant pill Dexatrim goes on the market. It is one of the first in a series of such drugs to come to market. Side effects such as stroke and heart attacks caused many of them to be removed from shelves.

1977—Liquid Diets Arrive

SlimFast becomes the first in a long line of "liquid" dietary staples. It advocates having a shake for breakfast and lunch, and then a sensible dinner. It is a grandparent of the "juicing" diet.

1978—Dieting in Scarsdale

Herman Tarnower, M.D., publishes *The Complete Scarsdale Medical Diet*. It is a high-protein, low-carb diet.

1979—Pritikin: Fat Is Out

The Pritikin Diet answers the trend of the high-protein, low-carb diets with a high-fiber, very-low-fat diet. Fat is your enemy.

1981—Back to Hollywood: Food Is Out

The Beverly Hills Diet recommends eating nothing but fruit for the first 10 days.

1985—Peas at Noon, Hamburgers at Night

Harvey and Marilyn Diamond publish *Fit for Life,* which prohibits complex carbs and protein from being eaten during the same meal.

1992—Atkins: Fat Is Back

Robert C. Atkins, M.D., publishes *Dr. Atkins' New Diet Revolution*, a high-protein, low-carb plan. Fat is your friend.

1995—Zone: Balance Is Back

The Zone Diet, which calls for a specific ratio of carbs, fat, and protein at each meal, ushered in the 40-30-30 ratio of carbs, fat, and protein.

1996—Blood Types Are In

Eat Right for Your Type by Peter J. D'Adamo paired diets with blood type.

2000—Macrobiotic Is Back

The Macrobiotic Diet is popularized by celebrities who prefer the restrictive Japanese plan based on whole grains and veggies.

2003—South Beach: "White Foods" Are Out

Miami doctor Arthur Agatston, M.D., publishes *The South Beach Diet*, seen as a more moderate version of Atkins. "White foods" (carbs) are off the menu.

2010—Paleo Is Back as Fantasy

The Paleo Diet, The Paleo Solution, and *The Primal Blueprint* books urge people to get in touch with their inner meat lover, ignoring the archeological evidence that early man also ate plants, vegetables, grains, and fruit.

Circa 2010—Gluten Is Out

With the rise in awareness of celiac disease and the popularity of *Wheat Belly, Grain Brain,* and Miley Cyrus, gluten has become the target of much hype and bad publicity.

Today—Take Your Pick

> Raw food diet
>
> Vegan—forgoing all animal products
>
> Vegetarian
>
> Anti-inflammatory diet of Dr. Andrew Weil
>
> Low-FODMAP
>
> Master Cleanse (lemonade diet)
>
> Juicing diet
>
> Gluten-free diet
>
> Atkins
>
> Weight Watchers
>
> The Whole30
>
> Orthorexia

Bottom Line: What goes around, comes around.

Resources

There are numerous resources available for people interested in more information on specific medical conditions. Any medical information obtained via national foundations, support groups, and/or professional groups should be used only for informational purposes. We are not endorsing its use for diagnostic or treatment purposes, which can only be obtained through appropriate medical and professional consultation.

The following listings contain contact information that is accurate at time of publication. Website addresses and links may change.

General Information

National Digestive Diseases Information
Clearinghouse (NDDIC)
A service of the National Institute of Diabetes and Digestive and
Kidney Diseases (NIDDK), National Institutes of Health
http://digestive.niddk.nih.gov/index.htm

United States National Library of Medicine

A service of the U.S. National Library of Medicine and the National Institutes of Health. Links to PubMed and MedlinePlus

www.nlm.nih.gov

www.nlm.nih.gov/medlineplus

Gluten Free Watchdog

A site that makes information on state-of-the-art testing of products for gluten available to the consumer

www.glutenfreewatchdog.org

Books

There are several medical, dietary, and lifestyle books that deal with different aspects of the gluten-free diet as well as the different conditions associated with its ingestion. This brief list contains publications mentioned in the text and others that provide background on the issues discussed.

Blaser, Martin J. *Missing Microbes*. New York: Henry Holt & Co., 2014.

Case, Shelley RD, R.D. *Gluten Free: The Definitive Resource Guide*. Regina, Saskatchewan, Canada: Case Nutrition Consulting, Inc., 2016.

Gershon, Michael D. *The Second Brain*. New York: HarperCollins, 1998.

Hillson, Beth. *Gluten-Free Makeovers*. Boston: Da Capo Lifelong Books, 2011.

Lieberman, Daniel E. *The Story of the Human Body*. New York: Pantheon Books, 2013.

Papagianni, Dimitra, and Michael A. Morse. *The Neanderthals Rediscovered*. London: Thames and Hudson Ltd., 2013.

Roberts, Annalise. *Gluten Free Baking Classics*. Surrey: Agate, 2008.

Scarlata, Kate. *The Complete Idiot's Guide to Eating Well with IBS (Idiot's Guides)*. New York: Penguin Group, 2010.

Support Groups

There are a number of support groups for disease-specific information and advice. Several focus on gluten-related issues.

Celiac Disease Foundation
Patient and physician education, advocacy and research
www.celiac.org

Gluten Intolerance Group
www.gluten.org

Beyond Celiac (formerly National Foundation for Celiac Awareness)
www.celiaccentral.org

American Diabetes Association
www.diabetes.org

Autism Science Foundation
www.autismsciencefoundation.org

Autism Speaks
www.autismspeaks.org

Arsenic and Mercury Guidelines

The Environmental Protection Agency (EPA) and FDA have limits on the amount of arsenic in drinking water (tap and bottled) of 10 micrograms per liter. The EPA in the past set a reference dose for inorganic arsenic exposure of .3 micrograms per kilogram of body weight per day. Rice-based foods may contain inorganic arsenic. Arsenic in rice appears to be very bioavailable.

To reduce arsenic in your diet:

- Cook rice in large amounts of water and discard the water after cooking.
- Choose white rice instead of brown rice. Arsenic is concentrated in the outer layer of rice, which is removed to make white rice.
- If you eat flour-based gluten-free foods, limit your rice intake (most gluten-free flour-based foods will contain varying amounts of rice flour).
- Choose corn, soybean, or quinoa pasta (gluten-free) instead of pastas made from rice. Some gluten-free pastas contain a mix of grains.

- Choose crackers made from corn, tapioca, or buckwheat instead of rice.
- Choose snacks made without rice—popcorn, cheese, hummus, yogurt, etc.
- Check the arsenic content of your water.
- Do not use rice bran (it has been tested and found to have high levels of arsenic).
- Limit products sweetened with rice syrup.
- Choose gluten-free cereals, pitas, and tortillas that do not contain rice.
- Choose quinoa and other gluten-free grains (millet, buckwheat, teff) instead of rice.

To reduce mercury in your diet:

- Avoid tilefish, shark, swordfish, and king mackerel.
- Limit consumption of white (albacore) tuna to 6 ounces a week.
- Choose lower-mercury fish, including shrimp, pollack, salmon, canned light tuna, tilapia, catfish, and cod.
- When eating fish caught from local streams, rivers, and lakes, follow fish advisories from local authorities. If advice isn't available, limit your total intake of such fish to 6 ounces a week and 1 to 3 ounces for children.
- Limit your rice intake. Mercury is another heavy metal that can be leached from ground water.

Label Guidelines for
Eating Gluten-Free

The following ingredients must be avoided by those with celiac disease:

- Wheat (in all its forms, including kamut, semolina, spelt/farro, triticale, bulgur, durum, einkorn, emmer, farina, atta/chapati flour)
- Oats (unless labeled gluten-free)
- Rye
- Barley (malt)
- Brewer's yeast

These additives in FDA-regulated foods are generally safe for those with celiac disease:

- Artificial color and flavor
- Baking powder
- Baking soda
- Caramel color
- Citric acid

- Dextrin
- Hydrolyzed soy protein
- Maltodextrin
- Modified food starch
- Mono- and diglycerides
- Monosodium glutamate
- Natural and artificial color and flavor
- Soy, soy protein
- Soy lecithin
- Vanilla, vanilla extract
- Vinegar (no malt vinegar)
- Whey

In USDA foods not labeled gluten-free, check for the following ingredients (and contact the manufacturer if necessary to confirm the product is gluten-free):

- Dextrin
- Starch, modified food starch

Scientific Articles and Studies

There are several celiac disease experts in most countries who publish in scientifically reputable journals on a variety of topics related to gluten, and their articles can be found on PubMed. The following is a listing of some of the more recent research on the topic.

Most of Dr. Green's articles are available through the website of the Celiac Disease Center at Columbia, www.celiacdiseasecenter.columbia.edu.

An abstract or summary of the following articles is also available on www.ncbi.nlm.nih.gov/pubmed.

Extraintestinal Manifestations of Coeliac Disease. Leffler DA, Green PH, Fasano A. *Nat Rev Gastroenterol Hepatol.* 2015 Aug 11.

Gluten Introduction, Breastfeeding, and Celiac Disease: Back to the Drawing Board. Lebwohl B, Murray JA, Verdú EF, Crowe SE, Dennis M, Fasano A, Green PH, Guandalini S, Khosla C. *Am J Gastroenterol.* 2015 Aug 11.

Attitudes Toward Genetic Testing for Celiac Disease. Roy A, Pallai M, Lebwohl B, Taylor AK, Green PH. *J Genet Couns.* 2015 Aug 2.

Protein Tyrosine Phosphatase PTPRS Is an Inhibitory Receptor on Human and Murine Plasmacytoid Dendritic Cells. Bunin A, Sisirak V, Ghosh HS, Grajkowska LT, Hou ZE, Miron M, Yang C, Ceribelli M, Uetani N, Chaperot L, Plumas J, Hendriks W, Tremblay ML, Häcker H, Staudt LM, Green PH, Bhagat G, Reizis B. *Immunity*. 2015 Aug 18;43(2):277–88.

Coeliac Disease: The Association Between Quality of Life and Social Support Network Participation. Lee AR, Wolf R, Contento I, Verdeli H, Green PH. *J Hum Nutr Diet*. 2015 Jul 21.

Cardiovascular Disease in Patients with Coeliac Disease: A Systematic Review and Meta-Analysis. Emilsson L, Lebwohl B, Sundström J, Ludvigsson JF. *Dig Liver Dis*. 2015 Jun 16.

Celiac Crisis in a 64-Year-Old Woman: An Unusual Cause of Severe Diarrhea, Acidosis, and Malabsorption. Mrad RA, Ghaddara HA, Green PH, El-Majzoub N, Barada KA. *ACG Case Rep J*. 2015 Jan 16;2(2):95–7.

Trends in Celiac Disease Research. Ciaccio EJ, Bhagat G, Lewis SK, Green PH. *Comput Biol Med*. 2015 Jun 5.

Blockers of Angiotensin Other Than Olmesartan in Patients with Villous Atrophy: A Nationwide Case-Control Study. Mårild K, Lebwohl B, Green PH, Murray JA, Ludvigsson JF. *Mayo Clin Proc*. 2015 Jun;90(6):730–7.

Distinct and Synergistic Contributions of Epithelial Stress and Adaptive Immunity to Functions of Intraepithelial Killer Cells and Active Celiac Disease. Setty M, Discepolo V, Abadie V, Kamhawi S, Mayassi T, Kent A, Ciszewski C, Maglio M, Kistner E, Bhagat G, Semrad C, Kupfer SS, Green PH, Guandalini S, Troncone R, Murray JA, Turner JR, Jabri B. *Gastroenterology*. 2015 May 19.

Suggestions for Automatic Quantitation of Endoscopic Image Analysis to Improve Detection of Small Intestinal Pathology in Celiac Disease Patients. Ciaccio EJ, Bhagat G, Lewis SK, Green PH. *Comput Biol Med*. 2015 Apr 24.

The Coeliac Stomach: Gastritis in Patients with Coeliac Disease. Lebwohl B, Green PH, Genta RM. *Aliment Pharmacol Ther*. 2015 Jul;42(2):180–7.

Risk of Neuropathy Among 28,232 Patients with Biopsy-Verified Celiac Disease. Thawani SP, Brannagan TH 3rd, Lebwohl B, Green PH, Ludvigsson JF. *JAMA Neurol*. 2015 Jul 1;72(7):806–11.

Celiac Disease. Green PH, Lebwohl B, Greywoode R. *J Allergy Clin Immunol.* 2015 May;135(5):1099–106.

Clinical Manifestations of Celiac Disease. Green PH, Krishnareddy S, Lebwohl B. *Dig Dis.* 2015;33(2):137–40.

Celiac Disease and the Forgotten 10%: The "Silent Minority." Lebwohl B. *Dig Dis Sci.* 2015 Jun;60(6):1517–8.

Abnormal Skeletal Strength and Microarchitecture in Women with Celiac Disease. Stein EM, Rogers H, Leib A, McMahon DJ, Young P, Nishiyama K, Guo XE, Lewis S, Green PH, Shane E. *J Clin Endocrinol Metab.* 2015 Jun;100(6):2347–53.

Cost Effectiveness of Routine Duodenal Biopsy Analysis for Celiac Disease During Endoscopy for Gastroesophageal Reflux. Yang JJ, Thanataveerat A, Green PH, Lebwohl B. *Clin Gastroenterol Hepatol.* 2015 Aug;13(8):1437–43.

Exploring the Strange New World of Non-Celiac Gluten Sensitivity. Lebwohl B, Leffler DA. *Clin Gastroenterol Hepatol.* 2015 Sep;13(9):1613–5.

Quantitative Image Analysis of Celiac Disease. Ciaccio EJ, Bhagat G, Lewis SK, Green PH. *World J Gastroenterol.* 2015 Mar 7;21(9):2577–81.

Increased Risk of Esophageal Eosinophilia and Eosinophilic Esophagitis in Patients with Active Celiac Disease on Biopsy. Jensen ET, Eluri S, Lebwohl B, Genta RM, Dellon ES. *Clin Gastroenterol Hepatol.* 2015 Aug;13(8):1426–31.

Larazotide Acetate for Persistent Symptoms of Celiac Disease Despite a Gluten-Free Diet: A Randomized Controlled Trial. Leffler DA, Kelly CP, Green PH, Fedorak RN, DiMarino A, Perrow W, Rasmussen H, Wang C, Bercik P, Bachir NM, Murray JA. *Gastroenterology.* 2015 Jun;148(7):1311–9.

Endoscopic Biopsy Technique in the Diagnosis of Celiac Disease: One Bite or Two? Latorre M, Lagana SM, Freedberg DE, Lewis SK, Lebwohl B, Bhagat G, Green PH. *Gastrointest Endosc.* 2015 May;81(5):1228–33.

Mucosal Healing and the Risk of Ischemic Heart Disease or Atrial Fibrillation in Patients with Celiac Disease; a Population-Based Study. Lebwohl B, Emilsson L, Fröbert O, Einstein AJ, Green PH, Ludvigsson JF. *PLoS One.* 2015 Jan 30;10(1):e0117529.

Increased Risk of Non-Alcoholic Fatty Liver Disease After Diagnosis of Celiac Disease. Reilly NR, Lebwohl B, Hultcrantz R, Green PH, Ludvigsson JF. *J Hepatol.* 2015 Jun;62(6):1405–11.

Mucosal Healing in Patients with Celiac Disease and Outcomes of Pregnancy: A Nationwide Population-Based Study. Lebwohl B, Stephansson O, Green PH, Ludvigsson JF. *Clin Gastroenterol Hepatol.* 2015 Jun;13(6):1111–7.

The Impact of Proton Pump Inhibitors on the Human Gastrointestinal Microbiome. Freedberg DE, Lebwohl B, Abrams JA. *Clin Lab Med.* 2014 Dec;34(4):771–85.

Seroprevalence of Celiac Disease Among United Arab Emirates Healthy Adult Nationals: A Gender Disparity. Abu-Zeid YA, Jasem WS, Lebwohl B, Green PH, ElGhazali G. *World J Gastroenterol.* 2014 Nov 14;20(42):15830–6.

Assessing Bowel Preparation Quality Using the Mean Number of Adenomas Per Colonoscopy. Hillyer GC, Lebwohl B, Rosenberg RM, Neugut AI, Wolf R, Basch CH, Mata J, Hernandez E, Corley DA, Shea S, Basch CE. *Therap Adv Gastroenterol.* 2014 Nov;7(6):238–46.

Sprue-Like Histology in Patients with Abdominal Pain Taking Olmesartan Compared with Other Angiotensin Receptor Blockers. Lagana SM, Braunstein ED, Arguelles-Grande C, Bhagat G, Green PH, Lebwohl B. *J Clin Pathol.* 2015 Jan;68(1):29–32.

Specific Nongluten Proteins of Wheat Are Novel Target Antigens in Celiac Disease Humoral Response. Huebener S, Tanaka CK, Uhde M, Zone JJ, Vensel WH, Kasarda DD, Beams L, Briani C, Green PH, Altenbach SB, Alaedini A. *J Proeome Res.* 2015 Jan 2;14(1):503–11.

Editorial: Sprue-Like Enteropathy Due to Olmesartan and Other Angiotensin Receptor Blockers—the Plot Thickens. Lebwohl B, Ludvigsson JF. *Aliment Pharmacol Ther.* 2014 Nov;40(10):1245–6.

Editorial: Mucosal Healing and Adherence to the Gluten-Free Diet in Coeliac Disease. Lebwohl B, Ludvigsson JF. *Aliment Pharmacol Ther.* 2014 Nov;40(10):1241–2.

The Missing Environmental Factor in Celiac Disease. Ludvigsson JF, Green PH. *N Engl J Med.* 2014 Oct 2;371(14):1341–3.

Use of Basis Images for Detection and Classification of Celiac Disease. Ciaccio EJ, Tennyson CA, Bhagat G, Lewis SK, Green PH. *Biomed Mater Eng.* 2014;24(6):1913–23.

Methods to Quantitate Videocapsule Endoscopy Images in Celiac Disease. Ciaccio EJ, Tennyson CA, Bhagat G, Lewis SK, Green PH. *Biomed Mater Eng.* 2014;24(6):1895–911.

Risk of Celiac Disease According to HLA Haplotype and Country. Lebwohl B, Green P. *N Engl J Med.* 2014 Sep 11;371(11):1073–4.

Dietary Supplement Use in Patients with Celiac Disease in the United States. Nazareth S, Lebwohl B, Tennyson CA, Simpson S, Greenlee H, Green PH. *J Clin Gastroenterol.* 2015 Aug;49(7):577–81.

Rates of Suboptimal Preparation for Colonoscopy Differ Markedly Between Providers: Impact on Adenoma Detection Rates. Mahadev S, Green PH, Lebwohl B. *J Clin Gastroenterol.* 2014 Aug 20.

Editorial: "Brain Fog" and Coeliac Disease—Evidence for Its Existence. Lebwohl B, Ludvigsson JF. *Aliment Pharmacol Ther.* 2014 Sep;40(5):565.

Olmesartan, Other Antihypertensives, and Chronic Diarrhea Among Patients Undergoing Endoscopic Procedures: A Case-Control Study. Greywoode R, Braunstein ED, Arguelles-Grande C, Green PH, Lebwohl B. *Mayo Clin Proc.* 2014 Sep;89(9):1239–43.

Isotretinoin Use and Celiac Disease: A Population-Based Cross-Sectional Study. Lebwohl B, Sundström A, Jabri B, Kupfer SS, Green PH, Ludvigsson JF. *Am J Clin Dermatol.* 2014 Dec;15(6):537–42.

Genome-Wide Association Study of Celiac Disease In North America Confirms FRMD4B as New Celiac Locus. Garner C, Ahn R, Ding YC, Steele L, Stoven S, Green PH, Fasano A, Murray JA, Neuhausen SL. *PLoS One.* 2014 Jul 7;9(7):e101428.

Diagnosis and Management of Adult Coeliac Disease: Guidelines from the British Society of Gastroenterology. Ludvigsson JF, Bai JC, Biagi F, Card TR, Ciacci C, Ciclitira PJ, Green PH, Hadjivassiliou M, Holdoway A, van Heel DA, Kaukinen K, Leffler DA, Leonard JN, Lundin KE, McGough N, Davidson M, Murray JA, Swift GL, Coeliac Disease Guidelines Development Group; British Society of Gastroenterology. Walker MM, Zingone F, Sanders DS; BSG *Gut.* 2014 Aug;63(8):1210–28.

How Often Do Hematologists Consider Celiac Disease in Iron-Deficiency Anemia? Results of a National Survey. Smukalla S, Lebwohl B, Mears JG, Leslie LA, Green PH. *Clin Adv Hematol Oncol.* 2014 Feb;12(2):100–5.

Development and Validation of a Clinical Prediction Score (the SCOPE Score) to Predict Sedation Outcomes in Patients Undergoing Endoscopic Procedures. Braunstein ED, Rosenberg R, Gress F, Green PH, Lebwohl B. *Aliment Pharmacol Ther.* 2014 Jul;40(1):72–82.

Utilizing HDL Levels to Improve Detection of Celiac Disease in Patients with Iron Deficiency Anemia. Abu Daya H, Lebwohl B, Smukalla S, Lewis SK, Green PH. *Am J Gastroenterol.* 2014 May;109(5):769–70.

Risk of Cutaneous Malignant Melanoma in Patients with Celiac Disease: A Population-Based Study. Lebwohl B, Eriksson H, Hansson J, Green PH, Ludvigsson JF. *J Am Acad Dermatol.* 2014 Aug;71(2):245–8.

Issues Associated with the Emergence of Coeliac Disease in the Asia–Pacific Region: A Working Party Report of the World Gastroenterology Organization and the Asian Pacific Association of Gastroenterology. Makharia GK, Mulder CJ, Goh KL, Ahuja V, Bai JC, Catassi C, Green PH, Gupta SD, Lundin KE, Ramakrishna BS, Rawat R, Sharma H, Sood A, Watanabe C, Gibson PR; World Gastroenterology Organization-Asia Pacific Association of Gastroenterology Working Party on Celiac Disease. *J Gastroenterol Hepatol.* 2014 Apr;29(4):666–77.

Lack of Serologic Evidence to Link IgA Nephropathy with Celiac Disease or Immune Reactivity to Gluten. Moeller S, Canetta PA, Taylor AK, Arguelles-Grande C, Snyder H, Green PH, Kiryluk K, Alaedini A. *PLoS One.* 2014 Apr 14;9(4):e94677.

No Association Between Biopsy-Verified Celiac Disease and Subsequent Amyotrophic Lateral Sclerosis—a Population-Based Cohort Study. Ludvigsson JF, Mariosa D, Lebwohl B, Fang F. *Eur J Neurol.* 2014 Jul;21(7):976–82.

Re: "Decreased Risk of Celiac Diseasei Patients with Helicobacter Pylori Colonization." The Authors Reply. Lebwohl B, Blaser MJ, Ludvigsson JF, Green PH, Rundle A, Sonnenberg A, Genta RM. *Am J Epidemiol.* 2014 May 15;179(10):1275–6.

Characteristics Associated with Suboptimal Bowel Preparation Prior to Colonoscopy: Results of a National Survey. Basch CH, Hillyer GC, Basch CE, Lebwohl B, Neugut AI. *Int J Prev Med.* 2014 Feb;5(2):233–7.

Prediction of Celiac Disease at Endoscopy. Barada K, Habib RH, Malli A, Hashash JG, Halawi H, Maasri K, Tawil A, Mourad F, Sharara AI, Soweid A, Sukkarieh I, Chakhachiro Z, Jabbour M, Fasano A, Santora D, Arguelles C, Murray JA, Green PH. *Endoscopy.* 2014 Feb;46(2):110–9.

Celiac Disease Is Diagnosed Less Frequently in Young Adult Males. Dixit R, Lebwohl B, Ludvigsson JF, Lewis SK, Rizkalla-Reilly N, Green PH. *Dig Dis Sci.* 2014 Jul;59(7):1509–12.

Persistent Mucosal Damage and Risk of Fracture in Celiac Disease. Lebwohl B, Michaëlsson K, Green PH, Ludvigsson JF. *J Clin Endocrinol Metab.* 2014 Feb;99(2):609–16.

Predictors of Persistent Villous Atrophy in Coeliac Disease: A Population-Based Study. Lebwohl B, Murray JA, Rubio-Tapia A, Green PH, Ludvigsson JF. *Aliment Pharmacol Ther.* 2014 Mar;39(5):488–95.

Characteristics of Patients Who Avoid Wheat and/or Gluten in the Absence of Celiac Disease. Tavakkoli A, Lewis SK, Tennyson CA, Lebwohl B, Green PH. *Dig Dis Sci.* 2014 Jun;59(6):1255–61.

Dermatitis herpetiformis: Clinical Presentations Are Independent of Manifestations of Celiac Disease. Krishnareddy S, Lewis SK, Green PH. *Am J Clin Dermatol.* 2014 Feb;15(1):51–6.

The Unfolding Story of Celiac Disease Risk Factors. Lebwohl B, Ludvigsson JF, Green PH. *Clin Gastroenterol Hepatol.* 2014 Apr;12(4):632–5.

Screening Colonoscopy Bowel Preparation: Experience in an Urban Minority Population. Basch CH, Basch CE, Wolf RL, Zybert P, Lebwohl B, Shmukler C, Neugut AI, Shea S. *Therap Adv Gastroenterol.* 2013 Nov;6(6):442–6.

Decreased Risk of Celiac Disease in Patients with *Helicobacter pylori* Colonization. Lebwohl B, Blaser MJ, Ludvigsson JF, Green PH, Rundle A, Sonnenberg A, Genta RM. *Am J Epidemiol.* 2013 Dec 15;178(12):1721–30.

Lack of Association Between Autism and Anti-GM1 Ganglioside Antibody. Moeller S, Lau NM, Green PH, Hellberg D, Higgins JJ, Rajadhyaksha AM, Alaedini A. *Neurology.* 2013 Oct 29;81(18):1640–1.

Use of Proton Pump Inhibitors and Subsequent Risk of Celiac Disease. Lebwohl B, Spechler SJ, Wang TC, Green PH, Ludvigsson JF. *Dig Liver Dis.* 2014 Jan;46(1):36–40.

Interest in Medical Therapy for Celiac Disease. Tennyson CA, Simpson S, Lebwohl B, Lewis S, Green PH. *Therap Adv Gastroenterol.* 2013 Sep;6(5):358–64.

Mucosal Healing and Risk For Lymphoproliferative Malignancy in Celiac Disease: A Population-Based Cohort Study. Lebwohl B, Granath F, Ekbom A, Smedby KE, Murray JA, Neugut AI, Green PH, Ludvigsson JF. *Ann Intern Med.* 2013 Aug 6;159(3):169–75.

Antibiotic Exposure and the Development of Coeliac Disease: A Nationwide Case-Control Study. Mårild K, Ye W, Lebwohl B, Green PH, Blaser MJ, Card T, Ludvigsson JF. *BMC Gastroenterol.* 2013 Jul 8;13:109.

Prevalence of Gluten-Free Diet Adherence Among Individuals Without Celiac Disease in the USA: Results from the Continuous National Health and Nutrition Examination Survey 2009–2010. DiGiacomo DV, Tennyson CA, Green PH, Demmer RT. *Scand J Gastroenterol.* 2013 Aug;48(8):921–5.

Markers of Celiac Disease and Gluten Sensitivity in Children with Autism. Lau NM, Green PH, Taylor AK, Hellberg D, Ajamian M, Tan CZ, Kosofsky BE, Higgins JJ, Rajadhyaksha AM, Alaedini A. *PLoS One.* 2013 Jun 18;8(6):e66155.

Post-Colonoscopy Recommendations after Inadequate Bowel Preparation: All in the Timing. Lebwohl B, Neugut AI. *Dig Dis Sci.* 2013 Aug;58(8):2135–7.

Celiac Disease Patients Presenting with Anemia Have More Severe Disease Than Those Presenting with Diarrhea. Abu Daya H, Lebwohl B, Lewis SK, Green PH. *Clin Gastroenterol Hepatol.* 2013 Nov;11(11):1472–7.

Men with Celiac Disease Are Shorter Than Their Peers in the General Population. Sonti R, Lebwohl B, Lewis SK, Abu Daya H, Klavan H, Aguilar K, Green PH. *Eur J Gastroenterol Hepatol.* 2013 Sep;25(9):1033–7.

Development and Validation of a Celiac Disease Quality of Life Instrument for North American Children. Jordan NE, Li Y, Magrini D, Simpson S, Reilly NR, Defelice AR, Sockolow R, Green PH. *J Pediatr Gastroenterol Nutr.* 2013 Oct;57(4):477–86.

Is Dietitian Use Associated with Celiac Disease Outcomes? Mahadev S, Simpson S, Lebwohl B, Lewis SK, Tennyson CA, Green PH. *Nutrients.* 2013 May 15;5(5):1585–94.

Celiac Disease in Patients with Type 1 Diabetes: Screening and Diagnostic Practices. Simpson SM, Ciaccio EJ, Case S, Jaffe N, Mahadov S, Lebwohl B, Green PH. *Diabetes Educ.* 2013 Jul-Aug;39(4):532–40.

Gastrointestinal Dysfunction in Autism: Parental Report, Clinical Evaluation, and Associated Factors. Gorrindo P, Williams KC, Lee EB, Walker LS, McGrew SG, Levitt P. *Autism Res.* 2012 Apr;5(2):101–8.

Rigid-Compulsive Behaviors Are Associated with Mixed Bowel Symptoms in Autism Spectrum Disorder. Peters B, Williams KC, Gorrindo P, Rosenberg D, Lee EB, Levitt P, Veenstra-VanderWeele J. *J Autism Dev Disord.* 2014 Jun;44(6).

Cognitive Impairment in Coeliac Disease Improves on a Gluten-Free Diet and Correlates with Histological and Serological Indices of Disease Severity. Lichtwark IT, Newnham ED, Robinson SR, Shepherd SJ, Hosking P, Gibson PR, Yelland GW. *Aliment Pharmacol Ther.* 2014 Jul;40(2):160–70.

Effects of a Gluten-Free Diet on Gut Microbiota and Immune Function in Healthy Adult Human Subjects. De Palma, Giada; Nadal, Inmaculada; Collado, Maria Carmen; Sanz, Yolanda. *The British Journal of Nutrition.* 102.8 (Oct 28, 2009): 1154–60.

Gluten Contamination of Commercial Oat Products in the United States. Trisha Thompson, M.S., R.D. *N Engl J Med.* 2004; 351:2021–2.

A Nationwide Population-Based Study on the Risk of Coma, Ketoacidosis and Hypoglycemia in Patients with Celiac Disease and Type 1 Diabetes. Kurien M, Mollazadegan K, Sanders DS, Ludvigsson JF. *Acta Diabetol.* 2015 Dec;52(6):1167–74.

Editorial: Adherence in Coeliac Disease—Those That Can Will and Those That Can't Won't (and Need Support)! Kurien M, Sanders DS. *Aliment Pharmacol Ther.* 2015 Oct;42(7):934–5.

Cost and Availability of Gluten-Free Food in the UK: In Store and Online. Burden M, Mooney PD, Blanshard RJ, White WL, Cambray-Deakin DR, Sanders DS. *Postgrad Med J.* 2015 Nov;91(1081):622–6.

Noncoeliac Gluten Sensitivity: A Diagnostic Dilemma. Branchi F, Aziz I, Conte D, Sanders DS. *Curr Opin Clin Nutr Metab Care.* 2015 Sep;18(5):508–14.

The Spectrum of Noncoeliac Gluten Sensitivity. Aziz I, Hadjivassiliou M, Sanders DS. *Nat Rev Gastroenterol Hepatol.* 2015 Sep;12(9):516–26.

Gastro-Oesophageal Reflux Symptoms and Coeliac Disease: No Role for Routine Duodenal Biopsy. Mooney PD, Evans KE, Kurien M, Hopper AD, Sanders DS. *Eur J Gastroenterol Hepatol.* 2015 Jun;27(6):692–7.

Support for Patients with Celiac Disease: A Literature Review. Ludvigsson JF, Card T, Ciclitira PJ, Swift GL, Nasr I, Sanders DS, Ciacci C. *United European Gastroenterol J.* 2015 Apr;3(2):146–59.

Psychological Morbidity of Celiac Disease: A Review of the Literature. Zingone F, Swift GL, Card TR, Sanders DS, Ludvigsson JF, Bai JC. *United European Gastroenterol J.* 2015 Apr;3(2):136–45.

The Gluten-Free Diet and Its Current Application in Coeliac Disease and *Dermatitis herpetiformis.* Ciacci C, Ciclitira P, Hadjivassiliou M, Kaukinen K, Ludvigsson JF, McGough N, Sanders DS, Woodward J, Leonard JN, Swift GL. *United European Gastroenterol J.* 2015 Apr;3(2):121–35.

Screening for Celiac Disease in the General Population and in High-Risk Groups. Ludvigsson JF, Card TR, Kaukinen K, Bai J, Zingone F, Sanders DS, Murray JA. *United European Gastroenterol J.* 2015 Apr;3(2):106–20.

Small-Bowel Capsule Endoscopy and Device-Assisted Enteroscopy for Diagnosis and Treatment of Small-Bowel Disorders: European Society of Gastrointestinal Endoscopy (ESGE) Clinical Guideline. Pennazio M, Spada C, Eliakim R, Keuchel M, May A, Mulder CJ, Rondonotti E, Adler SN, Albert J, Baltes P, Barbaro F, Cellier C, Charton JP, Delvaux M, Despott EJ, Domagk D, Klein A, McAlindon M, Rosa B, Rowse G, Sanders DS, Saurin JC, Sidhu R, Dumonceau JM, Hassan C, Gralnek IM. *Endoscopy.* 2015 Apr;47(4):352–76.

Prevalence of Idiopathic Bile Acid Diarrhea Among Patients with Diarrhea-Predominant Irritable Bowel Syndrome Based on Rome III Criteria. Aziz I, Mumtaz S, Bholah H, Chowdhury FU, Sanders DS, Ford AC. High *Clin Gastroenterol Hepatol.* 2015 Sep;13(9):1650–5.e2.

Systematic Review: Noncoeliac Gluten Sensitivity. Molina-Infante J, Santolaria S, Sanders DS, Fernández-Bañares F. *Aliment Pharmacol Ther.* 2015 May;41(9):807–20.

A Study Evaluating the Bidirectional Relationship Between Inflammatory Bowel Disease and Self-Reported Non-Celiac Gluten Sensitivity. Aziz I, Branchi F, Pearson K, Priest J, Sanders DS. *Inflamm Bowel Dis.* 2015 Apr;21(4):847–53.

The Rise and Fall of Gluten! Aziz I, Branchi F, Sanders DS. *Proc Nutr Soc.* 2015 Aug;74(3):221–6.

Editorial: Is a Histological Diagnosis Mandatory for Adult Patients with Suspected Coeliac Disease? Kurien M, Mooney PD, Sanders DS. *Aliment Pharmacol Ther.* 2015 Jan;41(1):146–7.

A No Biopsy Strategy for Adult Patients with Suspected Coeliac Disease: Making the World Gluten-Free. Kurien M, Ludvigsson JF, Sanders DS; authors of the BSG guidelines. *Gut.* 2015 Jun;64(6):1003–4.

Support for Patients with Celiac Disease: A Literature Review. Ludvigsson JF, Card T, Ciclitira PJ, Swift GL, Nasr I, Sanders DS, Ciacci C. *United European Gastroenterol J.* 2015 Apr;3(2):146–59.

Gastrointestinal Effects of Eating Quinoa (*Chenopodium quinoa Willd.*) in Celiac Patients. Zevallos VF, Herencia LI, Chang F, Donnelly S, Ellis HJ, Ciclitira PJ. *Am J Gastroenterol.* 2014 Feb;109(2):270–8.

Evaluation of the Safety of Ancient Strains of Wheat in Coeliac Disease Reveals Heterogeneous Small Intestinal T Cell Responses Suggestive of Coeliac Toxicity. Šuligoj T, Gregorini A, Colomba M, Ellis HJ, Ciclitira PJ. *Clin Nutr.* 2013 Dec;32(6):1043–9.

Celiac Disease: Management of Persistent Symptoms in Patients on a Gluten-Free Diet. Dewar DH, Donnelly SC, McLaughlin SD, Johnson MW, Ellis HJ, Ciclitira PJ. *World J Gastroenterol,* 2012 Mar 28;18(12):1348–56.

Pharmacotherapy and Management Strategies for Coeliac Disease. Donnelly SC, Ellis HJ, Ciclitira PJ. *Expert Opin Pharmacother.* 2011 Aug;12(11):1731–44.

Electrochemical Immunosensor for Detection of Celiac Disease Toxic Gliadin in Foodstuff. Nassef HM, Bermudo Redondo MC, Ciclitira PJ, Ellis HJ, Fragoso A, O'Sullivan CK. *Anal Chem.* 2008 Dec 1;80(23):9265–71.

Glossary

Affective disorders—Those disorders relating to moods, feelings, and/or attitudes.

Alleles—The different forms of a given gene.

Amylase—An enzyme secreted by the salivary glands and pancreas that breaks down starches (carbohydrates) into simple sugars.

Anaphylaxis—A sudden, severe systemic allergic reaction to a substance that causes inflammation in various parts of the body. Symptoms can be mild or potentially life threatening. It can affect the skin, blood pressure, breathing, and digestion.

Antibody—Antibodies are proteins secreted by cells of the immune system. They are found in the bloodstream and body tissues and protect the body from various foreign substances and infections. (See also *Immunoglobulin*.)

Antigen—Any foreign material that causes your immune system to produce antibodies against it.

Antigliadin antibodies (**AGA**)—A food antibody that targets the protein found in wheat.

Ataxia—A balance disturbance that affects motor control and coordination. It can affect limbs, body, speech, and eye movements and is also associated with degenerative diseases of the central nervous system.

Atherosclerosis—A hardening of the arteries due to the buildup of plaque, cholesterol, and other substances in artery walls

Bacteroides—A phylum of bacterium found in the GI tract and part of our microbiota.

Barrett's esophagus—An abnormality of the lining of the lower esophagus due to chronic reflux, considered premalignant.

Bifidobacteria—One of the dominant microbial populations of the intestinal tract.

Bile duct—The duct that connects the liver to the small intestine and enables bile to be released into the center of the duodenum.

Bile—A liver secretion that aids in the digestion of fats.

Bolus—A lump or mass. Used in two different contexts: A bolus of partially digested food is propelled from the stomach into the duodenum. Also as in a bolus of insulin that is the extra dose of short-acting insulin taken by a diabetic before a meal or snack to control or cover the glucose in the food.

Brush border—The microvilli or tiny "hairs" covering the villi of the small intestine that increase the absorptive area of the small intestine, and secrete specific enzymes that aid in digestion. When the microvilli are flattened or destroyed, both of these functions are impaired or halted.

Cerebral calcification—A calcium deposit in the brain.

Chyme—A soupy solution formed in the stomach consisting of food, gastric juices, enzymes, and saliva.

Clostridium difficile (*C. difficile* **or** *C. diff*)—A bacterium found in the intestines. This is regarded as one of the superbugs.

Coeliac disease—A spelling of celiac disease commonly used outside the U.S.

Collagenous sprue—A lesion within the small intestine in which inflammatory cells lay down a thickened band of fibrous tissue. It can occur in any type of villous atrophy including celiac disease and intestinal inflammatory disease caused by the drug olmesartan.

Colon—The lower end of the digestive tract.

Cytokines—Protein "messengers" produced by inflammatory cells to respond to infections, which increase the inflammatory response. They are released by cells to affect the behavior of other cells.

Dementia—Disorientation and/or impairment of mental processes caused by disease, old age, trauma, stroke, or unknown factors. The definition of Alzheimer's dementia is different from that of dementia.

Dendric cells—A highly specialized white blood cell found in the skin, mucosa, and lymph tissues that initiates an immune response.

Dermatitis herpetiformis (DH)—An extremely itchy, blistering skin condition that is caused by IgA deposits in the layers of the skin. If you have a definitive diagnosis of DH, you have celiac disease.

Diverticula—Small sacs protruding from the intestinal wall that can occur anywhere in the GI tract. Most often encountered in the colon.

Dysbiosis—An imbalance or disruption, e.g., of the intestinal microbiota.

Dysphagia—Difficulty swallowing.

Electrolytes—Minerals in your blood and other body fluids that carry an electric charge. Electrolytes affect the amount of water in your body, the acidity of your blood (pH), your muscle function, and other important processes.

Emulsification—The process through which fats are broken into small particles with a surface area that can unite or bind with water in order to pass through the intestinal wall. An emulsifying agent such as phospholipids keeps the droplets from reforming back into larger drops. This is the main function of bile.

Endoscopy—A minimally invasive procedure during which a small tube with a built-in camera is introduced into the body either through the mouth, colon, or airway. It can be used to take pictures or take tissue samples (biopsies), remove foreign bodies, and perform other therapeutic maneuvers.

Enteropathy—Any inflammatory disease of the small intestine characterized by villous atrophy.

Eosinophilic esophagitis (EOE)—An inflammation of the esophagus that causes food to "stick" and trouble swallowing.

Eosinophils—A type of white blood cell often present in immune reactions and allergies.

Epithelium—A grouping of cells that make up most of the surfaces of the body and line the GI tract.

Erythrocyte sedimentation rate (ESR)—A blood test to determine levels of inflammation in the body.

Etiology—The origins and causes of a disease.

Firmicutes—A phylum of bacteria found in the GI tract and part of our microbiota, includes other classes of bacteria such as *Lactobacillus, Streptococcus,* and *Clostridium.*

FODMAPs—Fermentable oligosaccharides, disaccharides, monosaccharides, and polyols. The carbohydrates found in many plants, vegetables, and fruits.

Fumonisin—A mycotoxin or environmental toxin that is produced by various fungi and molds. It occurs in the field or during storage, mainly in corn.

Gastric acid—The highly effective—and highly corrosive—acid that helps to digest the food in the stomach. It is also protective against infections.

Gastroenteritis—Inflammation of the digestive tract by food or pathogens, resulting in gastrointestinal symptoms.

Gastroparesis—Delayed emptying of the stomach. May be caused by decreased intestinal motility due to diabetes, scleroderma, or celiac disease.

GERD—Gastroesophageal reflux disease.

Gestational diabetes—A type of diabetes that occurs during pregnancy and usually resolves once the baby is born.

GI—Gastrointestinal.

Gliadin—The alcohol-soluble fraction of gluten found in wheat; the most studied portion in celiac disease, but not necessarily the only toxic fraction in grains.

Globus—The sensation of a lump in the throat, a common symptom of GERD or anxiety.

Glucocorticoid—A class of steroid hormones secreted by the adrenal glands in response to signals from the brain. They mobilize and replenish energy stores.

Gluten—The storage protein of wheat. Essentially, the portion of wheat flour that makes it "sticky." The gluten fraction that is most studied in celiac disease is called gliadin, but there are other proteins that chemically resemble gliadin in rye (secalins) and barley (hordeins). These proteins are not strictly glutens, but are generally included in the term.

Hiatal hernia—A condition where part of the stomach pushes through the diaphragm into the chest cavity. It is due to an enlargement of the opening in the diaphragm through which the esophagus passes.

Histamine receptor type 2 (H2RA) inhibitors—An acid reducer for healing ulcers and GERD; available in prescription and nonprescription form, e.g., Tagamet, Zantac, Pepcid.

Histamines—Substances released into tissues and the bloodstream that produce the symptoms of allergy including inflammation, itching, swelling, etc.

Homeostasis—Regulation of metabolic functions so that their processes remain stable and constant.

Hordeins—See *Gluten.*

Human leukocyte antigens (HLA)—Proteins that sit on the surface of white blood cells that play an important role in the immune system by reacting with foreign substances. These proteins are genetically determined, and every person receives one set from each parent.

Hyperglycemia—High blood glucose levels commonly seen in diabetics who do not have enough, or any, insulin that is required to metabolize the glucose for use by the body. Usually apparent after a meal.

Hypoglycemia—Low blood glucose levels commonly observed when too much insulin is administered, or too little food eaten to cover the insulin given.

Ileitis—An inflammation of the ileum.

Immunoglobulin (Ig)—Proteins secreted by specific white blood cells protecting the body against bacteria and viruses.

Immunoglobulin A (IgA)—The antibodies secreted by plasma cells into the lining of the GI tract, tissues, and bloodstream that act locally in the lining or on the surface to disinfect our ingested food. Other classes of immunoglobulins include IgE, IgM, IgD and IgE.

Inflammatory bowel disease (IBD)—Chronic inflammation of the digestive tract of unclear cause. Includes both ulcerative colitis and Crohn's disease.

Inflammatory markers—Tests used to measure the levels of inflammation in the body; e.g., C-reactive protein (CRP), Erythrocyte sedimentation rate (ESR).

Insulin-dependent diabetes mellitus (IDDM)—Also known as type 1 diabetes or juvenile-onset diabetes. Characterized by the decreased or total absence of insulin.

Irritable bowel syndrome (IBS)—Any persistent condition with diarrhea and/

or constipation, gas, and abdominal pain that is not explained by other known diseases. There are strict criteria—the Rome criteria—that define the functional bowel disorders that include IBS, dyspepsia, functional bloating, and constipation.

Lactase—The enzyme secreted by the brush border of the small intestine that digests milk products. It is available commercially to treat lactase deficiency.

Lactose intolerance—A condition where lactase is not produced by the small intestine. Secondary lactose intolerance can occur when the brush border of the small intestine is damaged or destroyed and unable to produce the enzyme.

Lactulose—A nonmetabolized sugar.

Lipase(s)—The group of enzymes that break down fats into smaller and smaller components so they are able to be absorbed by the body. It is mainly secreted by the pancreas, but also by salivary glands (lingual lipase) that starts to digest fats in the stomach.

Lumen—The central, hollow portion of the digestive tube that is the site for the majority of digestive action.

Lupus or systemic lupus erythematosus (SLE)—An autoimmune disease in which the immune system attacks the various tissues within the body, leading to organ damage and dysfunction.

Mannitol—A nonmetabolized sugar.

Microbial antigen—Antigens are proteins that sit on the surface of a pathogen (any bacteria, virus, etc., that can cause disease) and causes the body to mount an immune response. The immune system produces antibodies that destroy the pathogen.

Microscopic colitis—An autoimmune inflammatory condition in the colon that may be associated with celiac disease. It is characterized by diarrhea, but no infection, and can vary in severity. It is diagnosed by biopsy.

Microvilli—The tiny hairlike projections lining each villus that further increase its absorptive potential.

Mucosa—The surface or superficial lining of the wall of the intestine. The mucosa consists of the epithelial (single) cell layer, the lamina propria, and a muscle layer.

Nerve conduction studies—Tests for nerve damage in which signals are run through nerve paths to determine if the nerve is functioning properly (i.e., conducting the signal and eliciting an appropriate response).

Neuropathy—A condition caused by the inflammation of nerves, resulting in altered sensation, weakness, or an array of other symptoms.

Olmesartan—A blood pressure medication that can cause a severe sprue-like disease. Patients may be told they have refractory celiac disease.

Orthorexia nervosa—A food disorder where people eliminate one food after another in the belief that the foods are "unhealthy," to the point of malnutrition.

Parathyroid hormone (PTH)—The hormone responsible for maintaining normal levels of calcium in the bloodstream. PTH increases the resorption of bone, causing calcium to be released into the bloodstream and the kidneys to retain calcium in the body. It also stimulates the activation of vitamin D that increases the intestinal absorption of calcium.

Parenteral nutrition (PN)—Feeding a person intravenously, bypassing the usual process of eating and digestion. The person receives nutrients such as glucose, amino acids, lipids, and added vitamins and dietary minerals.

Paresthesia—A burning, tingling, or prickling sensation that is usually felt in different parts of the body. The sensation is usually described as tingling or numbness, skin crawling, or itching.

Pediatric autoimmune neuropsychiatric disorders associated with streptococcal infections (PANDAS)—A subset of children with obsessive compulsive disorder (OCD) and/or tic disorders whose symptoms appear to be related to a streptococcus infection.

Pepsin—An enzyme secreted by the stomach that breaks down proteins. Part of a category of enzymes that break down protein.

Peptidases—A group of enzymes, such as pepsin, that breaks down proteins into smaller amino acid units.

Peptide bonds—The molecular bond that binds two amino acids.

Peripheral neuropathies—Numbness and/or tingling in the hands, face, and feet because of damaged peripheral nerves.

Peristalsis—The undulating contraction of the wall of the digestive tract that moves food down the digestive tube.

Proton pump inhibitors (PPIs)—A group of drugs whose main action is a pronounced and long-lasting reduction of gastric acid production.

Proximal intestine—The upper portion of the small intestine that includes the duodenum and the upper jejunum.

Rhinitis—Inflammation of the nasal membranes characterized by sneezing, nasal congestion, itching, and runny nose. Seasonal allergy.

Rotavirus—The most common cause of severe diarrhea among infants and young children.

Salivary glands—The mucous glands in and around the mouth that supply saliva to aid in swallowing and digestion.

Scleroderma—The thickening and scarring of certain tissues. It may involve skin, intestine, lungs or kidneys, and the heart. The effects depend on the organ involved.

Selective serotonin reuptake inhibitors (SSRIs) or serotonin-specific reuptake inhibitors—A class of drugs that block a receptor that reabsorbs serotonin, making more of it chemically available. Serotonin messaging is known to influence mood and pain perception.

Serologies—Blood tests. Serum (blood) is drawn and analyzed. Physicians can request specific panels (tests).

Serotonin (5-hydroxytryptamine [5-HT])—A biological base that functions as a neurotransmitter in the body.

Small intestine bacterial overgrowth (SIBO)—A disease characterized by an increase in the small intestine of bacteria that normally inhabit the colon. The bacteria cause poor fat and carbohydrate (sugar) absorption. The bacteria also use vitamin B12 for their own growth, causing B12 deficiency in the body.

Soluble—Able to dissolve in water. (See *Emulsification*.)

Sphincter—A muscle that acts as a break or valve. The esophageal and pyloric sphincter muscles control the entrance of food into the stomach and its exit into the duodenum, respectively. Spasms and/or malfunctions of these sphincters can be extremely painful and cause digestive problems.

Spruce—A tree.

Sprue—A syndrome in which there is an inflammatory disease of the intestines with villous atrophy that results in malabsorption (enteropathy). Celiac disease was formerly called celiac sprue in the U.S. It is currently used to define enteropathies such as tropical sprue, olmesartan enteropathy, and undefined sprue.

Stricture—An abnormal narrowing of a bodily passage (as from inflammation, cancer, or the formation of scar tissue).

Sucrase—Enzyme that breaks down sugars into glucose.

Synapsin—A protein found in the brain that regulates neurotransmitter release.

T-cells—A type of white blood cell that has various roles in the immune system, such as identifying specific foreign substances in the body; activating and deactivating other immune cells. A category of T-cells (CD4+ cells) plays a role in celiac disease.

Tenesmus—The feeling that more stool is there when, in fact, the feces are liquid and have been fully voided. A common condition in acute diarrhea.

Tissue transglutaminase (tTG)—An enzyme found in every tissue of the body that joins proteins together. It reacts with gliadin, setting off the chain of reactions that destroys the villi of the small intestine in celiac disease.

Toxoplasmosis—A parasitic disease caused by *Toxoplasma gondii* that occurs through infected meat; ingesting water, soil, or food that has come in contact with infected animal fecal matter (commonly household cats); or through transmission from an infected mother to her fetus during pregnancy.

tTG—See *Tissue transglutaminase*.

Type 1 Diabetes (IDDM)—See *Insulin-dependent diabetes mellitus*.

Type 2 Diabetes (NIDDM)—A condition where the pancreas cannot make enough insulin or does not use insulin properly (insulin resistance). Glucose builds up in the blood instead of being metabolized into the cells of the body.

Vagus nerve—A nerve that extends from the brain stem to the gut and commands unconscious body processes such as digestion.

Villi—Small projections lining the wall of the small intestine that greatly increase its absorptive power; they are lined with epithelial cells covered in microvilli that absorb nutrients.

Villus atrophy—The inflammation and eventual flattening (loss) of the villi of the small intestine resulting in a decreased surface for absorption.

Acknowledgments

This book evolved over the past few years, nurtured by the inter-disciplinary environment that research into celiac disease and the overall effect of gluten on the body requires. We would like to thank everyone we have worked and collaborated with over the past number of years, but some deserve a special mention for providing the energy and focus needed to explore this topic.

My colleagues in the Celiac Center, Drs. Alaedini, Bhagat, Krisndreddy, Lebwohl, Lewis, and Reilly continue to inspire me. Also, I thank my family—Marise and my beautiful daughters, Alanya and Isabella—for their support. In addition, the patients and friends of the Celiac Disease Center at Columbia University, upon whom we depend so much for supporting all our activities.

—Peter Green, M.D.

This book found shape and inspiration in each and every narrative shared with me over the past few years by family, students, patients, and friends. I am particularly indebted to those friends who brainstormed titles that nurtured the writing process as well as the writer. And very special thanks to my daughter, Rebecca Jones, Ph.D., whose understanding of the social brain was fundamental to clearing up misconceptions about gluten's role on and in the brain. And always, my family, especially David, deserves the deepest thanks for their endless patience and humor as gut disorders became the main topic of conversation at dinner.

—Rory Jones, M.S.

Finally, we both want to express special thanks to:

Our editor, Jennifer Civiletto, who patiently, tirelessly, and ferociously championed this book from its conceptual infancy, and expertly guided it with a steady hand to completion; Faith Hamlin, our agent, who knew that gluten was ready for its close-up and shepherded us as well as the book into print. Last, we both want to thank the many patients and friends who so generously gave us their time, insights, and opinions—and openly shared personal and often difficult stories about gluten and gluten-related disorders. We remain impressed by their resilience and desire to help others by sharing their medical journeys. This book is for you, and for the many people still making the journey to diagnosis.

Index

hookworms, 277
hormones, 139–40
Human Microbiome Project (HMP), 306
hygiene hypothesis, 21–22, 227

IBD. *See* inflammatory bowel disease
IBS. *See* irritable bowel syndrome
IDDM. *See* insulin-dependent diabetes
    mellitus
identity, 264–65
IgA, 55, 169–71
IgE, 56
IgG, 56, 170–71, 246
    antigliadin, 180
immune system
    environmental factors, 22–23
    in IBD, 196–97
    microbiome in, 91
    rotavirus and gluten in, 135–36
immunoglobulin primer, 55–56
immunosuppressants, 127–28
immunotherapy, 228
ImmusanT, 275–76
impulse control, 263
infant feeding, 163
inflammation, 98
    brain fog and, 257
    in celiac disease, 157
    cell responses in, 143–45
    definition, 142
    in GI tract, 141, 143
    heat changes in, 142–43
    intestinal permeability and, 150–51
    systemic, 145–46, 160
inflammatory bowel disease (IBD), 30,
    78–79, 194
    causes of, 196–99
    celiac disease and, 200
    definition, 195
    diagnosis of, 199
    diet for, 199–200

environmental factors, 198–99
genetics of, 196–99
immune responses in, 196–97
microbiome in, 197–98
smoking and, 198
treatment of, 199–200
insects, 100–101
insulin-dependent diabetes mellitus
    (IDDM), 80, 215–16
    carbohydrates and, 221–22
    celiac disease and, 220–21
    gluten and, 217
    screening, 218–20
intestinal permeability
    alterations in, 150
    autism and, 151–52
    inflammation and, 150–51
    inhibition of, 274
    microbiome and, 151
    tests for, 148–49
intestinal wall, 69
irritable bowel syndrome (IBS), 10, 30,
    83, 138
    brain-gut signal problems in, 188–89
    causes of, 186–89
    classifications, 184
    definition, 183–84
    diet for, 187, 191–92
    gate theory, 189–90
    genetics, 187
    gluten-free diet and, 14
    medication for, 190–91
    mental health and, 192
    microbiome and, 187–88
    post-infective, 188
    probiotics for, 192
    Rome III criteria, 185–86
    serotonin for, 191

lactase, 88, 272
Lactobacillus, 43